The
28-Day
GUT
Health Plan

**Lose Weight and Feel Better
from the Inside**

Jacqueline Whitehart

Thorsons

For Andy and the kids ... who are
always putting up with my experiments.

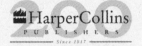

Thorsons
An imprint of HarperCollins*Publishers*
1 London Bridge Street,
London SE1 9GF
www.harpercollins.co.uk

1 3 5 7 9 10 8 6 4 2

Text © Jacqueline Whitehart 2017

Jacqueline Whitehart asserts her moral right to be identified
as the author of this work.

A catalogue record for this book is available from the British Library.

ISBN: 978-0-00-826891-6
EB ISBN: 978-0-00-826892-3

Printed and bound in Great Britain by CPI Group (UK) Ltd, Croydon

This book features weight-loss techniques which may not be suitable for
everyone. You should always consult with a qualified medical practitioner
before starting any weight-loss programme, or if you have any concerns about
your health. This book is not tailored to individual requirements or needs
and its contents are solely for general information purposes. It should not be
taken as professional or medical advice or diagnosis. The activities detailed in
this book should not be used as a substitute for any treatment or medication
prescribed or recommended to you by a medical practitioner. The author and
the publishers do not accept any responsibility for any adverse effects that may
occur as a result of the use of the suggestions or information herein. If you feel
that you are experiencing adverse effects after embarking on any weight-loss
programme, including the type described in this book, it is imperative that you
seek medical advice. Results may vary from individual to individual.

MIX
Paper from
responsible sources
FSC™ C007454

FSC™ is a non-profit international organisation established to promote
the responsible management of the world's forests. Products carrying the
FSC label are independently certified to assure consumers that they come
from forests that are managed to meet the social, economic and
ecological needs of present and future generations,
and other controlled sources.

Find out more about HarperCollins and the environment at
www.harpercollins.co.uk/green

The
28-Day
GUT
Health Plan

Jacqueline Whitehart is an expert health-food writer and best-selling cookery author.

With a practical and light-hearted approach, Jacqueline's books are full of helpful tips and advice, and are packed with her own fresh, healthy and delicious recipes.

Jacqueline is a busy working mum from Yorkshire who writes from the heart and from personal experience. She's not perfect, or a perfectionist; her down-to-earth approach to dieting and cooking speaks directly to her many readers, and she's always happy to answer any questions her readers may have.

Jacqueline's recipes are easy to follow with simple, readily available ingredients.

Jacqueline writes regularly on her blog, www.52recipes.co.uk, and has a weekly free-recipe newsletter.

CONTENTS

Part 1

FEEL BETTER FROM
THE INSIDE

INTRODUCTION

Do you get that Christmas dinner feeling every day of the week? Does your weight seem unaffected by what you eat and how often you exercise? Do you sometimes feel drained and bloated after a meal? Do you get bouts of spotty skin even though you're way past being a teenager? Does your stomach sometimes keep you awake at night?

Talking about our gut-health problems is a taboo subject for many of us. If you'd been up most of the night with stomach pains, would you mention it to your friend over coffee the next day? Would you mention your loose bowels at the school gates? Of course not. We keep the pain and anxiety well hidden. And if the pain and symptoms just get worse year on year, do we complain? No, we just get on with it and learn to manage the symptoms.

If you want weight loss, a flat stomach and a healthy digestion then let me steer you in the right direction. I challenge you to follow the 28-Day Gut-Health Plan. In four weeks, you'll lose weight – up to 3kg (7lb) – and it will all come off your tummy. You'll banish food cravings and restore the healthy bacteria in your gut. You'll take the first steps towards permanent weight loss, a healthier digestive system and a fitter old age.

What's more, with over 80 delicious recipes tailored to the programme, you'll find the plan to be both simple and tasty.

There are some really useful quizzes and trackers in the book and if you'd like them in a printable and reusable format, they are all available (at no cost) via **www.52recipes.co.uk/28G**

Finally, I'd like to say that I'm always here to answer your gut-health questions and help you overcome your personal hurdles. You can contact me by email at **j@52recipes.co.uk** or get in touch via **52DietRecipes** on Facebook or Twitter.

Yours,

Jacqueline

Jacqueline Whitehart

IS THE 28-DAY GUT-HEALTH PLAN FOR YOU?

Do you suffer occasional symptoms of gut sensitivity – bloating, gas, cramps or loose bowels? Do these symptoms appear quite randomly yet you can't tie them down to a particular foodstuff? Perhaps you suspect you might be intolerant to some foods but sometimes you can eat them without suffering any problems. The good news is that this plan can help you pinpoint the level of your food intolerances, reduce the symptoms and feel better and finally slowly reintroduce the food.

> **Severe Food Allergies**
> If you have a severe food allergy, such as nut or egg allergy, or suffer from coeliac disease then you should be following expert treatment. **This book is absolutely no substitute for professional medical advice.** The book can still be used to find other intolerances as long as you first seek expert medical advice.

If your weight loss has stalled (or hasn't even got going), then your gut could be holding you back. Your digestive system is like your second brain, telling you what to eat and when. When those signals get confused because your gut is a bit toxic (sorry for the bad news), then it tells you to eat when you're not hungry and gives you irresistible cravings. We're going to give your gut a deep clean and find out the foods your gut likes and the ones it struggles with. As a result, your cravings will disappear and you will naturally lose weight. It's not uncommon for someone following the gut-health programme (but not thinking about weight loss) to easily lose half a stone.

Cutting out trigger foods also forces us to cook more real food. Do you believe your ready meal doesn't contain gas-inducing veg? Wrong. It's in the stock. Think your cereal bar is good for you? Wrong. It contains at least twenty ingredients including five kinds of sugar or sweetener.

But don't worry. I know you don't want to spend hours in the kitchen, which is why I've included a whole section of easy and delicious recipes for you to try. My recipes are always fresh and simple, use common ingredients and have been tried and tested by me. All those faffy bits that restaurant chefs like to add to make their food look beautiful (but take half a day to prepare) ... they're not in my kitchen.

Onions and garlic are two of the more common causes of a sensitive belly. They are potent, gassy vegetables and even the tiniest amount can set many people off. I'll introduce you to a new cheap and easy-to-get-hold-of spice that you've probably never even heard of. Add a pinch of this to a dish to add natural onion flavour, without the tummy consequences – and without the chopping! What is it? You'll have to keep reading to find out!

Gut sensitivity affects as many as 10 to 15 per cent of people in the UK and that figure is rising. And that doesn't even include the thousands – perhaps even millions – of people with mild or occasional issues who just battle on and never visit the doctor or discuss it with anyone.

What I'd like to show you in this book is a way to get to grips with the causes of your gut-health problems. For just one month, we'll cut out possible trigger foods and introduce them again in a controlled fashion. You'll get your own personalized guide to foods you can eat with no problems, foods you can eat in moderation and foods to avoid.

The trigger food groups that we'll be looking at are: milk, red meat, nightshade (such as tomatoes and chillies), gassy vegetables and wheat.

Please don't think, 'That's it. You're telling me not to drink milk or eat bread ever again.' First of all, it is rare to be intolerant to both wheat and milk. And even if you find foods that you are intolerant to, you'll hopefully still be able to eat them in small quantities. You'll know how to choose the right foods for you. I'll give you the tools to help you make your own choices. It's like drinking alcohol. We all know that it gives us a hangover the next morning, but sometimes we do it anyway. You might find that tomatoes give you a rotten tummy ache, but occasionally you'll think it's a price worth paying.

A LITTLE BIT ABOUT DIFFERENT GUT SENSITIVITIES

One of the things that you quickly find when exploring gut sensitivities is that no two people are the same. How we react to certain foods and how our digestive systems behave is unique to us. Yet the mechanism is the same for everyone. And the root causes of all digestive issues are the same: inflammation of the gut lining, foods not being digested properly and the aptly titled 'leaky gut'.

In this book, I'll look at the root causes of digestive issues and explain how this can lead to IBS-like symptoms: stomach cramps and bloating and also to inflammation throughout our body. Frequent headaches, sinus pain and achy joints can all be linked back to our digestion.

HOW DOES THE 28-DAY GUT-HEALTH PLAN WORK?

The 28-Day Gut-Health Plan is a unique and simple programme that anyone can follow. With a scientific basis, down-to-earth advice and delicious recipes, **The Gut-Health Plan** delivers wellness, weight loss and a healthier gut.

The plan acknowledges that there are five common food triggers, as I've already mentioned – wheat, milk, nightshade, red meat and gassy vegetables – the cause of over 95 per cent of digestive difficulties. We rest the gut for a week then introduce each trigger individually on a three-day cycle to come up with a detailed plan of your own personal sensitivities.

The plan starts with a simple gut assessment to help you work out 'what's up'. You then follow a cycle of rest and food trials for the twenty-eight-day period, while recording your progress in a **Gut-Health Diary**. Plus you'll get my own personal brand of enthusiasm, advice and dedication to help you every step of the way.

At the end of the plan, as well as feeling better, having a flatter stomach and losing weight, you'll complete a **28-Day Review**. The review is designed to be your 'take-away' from the programme, with a simple checklist of what to eat and what to avoid for your own personal gut health.

We can't fix decades of 'food on the run' and 'processed food mania' in just one month. But we can help you make significant and noticeable changes in just four weeks. And with the tools that this programme provides, you can make better choices and continue to improve your gut in the long term.

We start in the **Rest and Restore Phase**, also known as the R&R phase, by cutting out damaging trigger foods. It can be limited but not boring with all the delicious recipes I have created for you to try. The diet is also low in sugar and as you will be avoiding processed food and eating three balanced meals a day, you will naturally lose weight and feel better.

Don't worry if you feel more bloated or your symptoms get worse over the first week. You are asking your body to do an awful lot. In fact the first week is really about building up the good bacteria and strengthening the gut so you are ready to start afresh in week two. If at any stage you hit a blip and feel your gut health deteriorating, put yourself back on the R&R programme.

Then over the following three weeks, you test each problem food individually, recording any gut consequences as you go. In this way, you build up a detailed picture of your own personal sensitivities.

WHAT'S WRONG WITH MY GUT?

An imbalanced digestive system is like a polluted river. It's grey and clogged with blockages. Years and years of pollution mean that the river is clogged up and the fish are few and far between.

Your gut lining is like a riverbank, muddy and bulging. The food you eat is like the water running through the river: it chugs along slowly, getting stuck and polluted. The fish are the good bacteria that have been killed off by years of 'food on the run'.

During the 28-Day Gut-Health Plan, we are going to cut out all the pollution – the junk foods and trigger foods – so that the river runs clear. We are going to reintroduce the 'fish' by adding probiotics to our diet. Then our gut will be strong again, and with a strong, healthy gut, the whole body is healthy and renewed.

COMMON GUT PROBLEMS

The symptoms of an unhealthy gut include bloating, gas, cramps, food sensitivities and aches and pains.

If these symptoms affect your daily life severely, this is classed as a medical problem and people are often diagnosed by their doctors as suffering from IBS. But the majority of us haven't reached that level. We're struggling on, just managing, and yet slowly the symptoms become more frequent and gut health becomes more of a worry.

The plan aims to reduce your symptoms and helps you learn what foods you should avoid, what foods you can have in moderation and the foods of which you can eat as much as you like.

The symptoms we are hoping to address are:

1. Stomach cramps
2. Bloating and swelling of your stomach
3. Diarrhoea
4. Constipation
5. Excessive Wind

THE PATH TO IBS

The five symptoms – stomach cramps, bloating, diarrhoea, constipation and excessive wind – that are classed as gut-health symptoms are also the symptoms of IBS. Whether you have IBS or not is simply a matter of severity. There is no test that you pass or fail for IBS; it is just a question of how your symptoms affect your daily life. If you get severe stomach cramps overnight then this means that you don't sleep well and your whole life is affected. This would be IBS. But occasional symptoms are annoying and we tend to just pick ourselves up and get on with it. The trouble is, year on year, your symptoms will slowly and almost imperceptibly get worse. You learn to manage them better, not complaining and just carrying on.

'Whatever stage you are at, this programme aims to reduce your symptoms by a significant and measurable amount.'

The easiest way to discover more about the health of your gut is to use the **Initial Gut Assessment Quiz** (see page 25). This gives you a gut-health score on a scale of 1 to 10 and helps you to answer the question: 'How bad is it?' If you want to see the progress in your gut health during the programme you can take the quiz again at the end of the plan and see by how much your score has reduced.

The aim of this plan is to reduce your symptoms and hopefully get rid of some of them entirely. You will gain a deeper understanding of your body and its sensitivities, so you are less likely to trigger them. If you find foods that you are sensitive to, don't worry too much as you will be able to eat them in moderation later on. Just in smaller quantities and less frequently.

DO YOU HAVE A 'LEAKY GUT'?

What is a leaky gut?
A leaky gut affects the whole body. It's caused by sections of the gut, normally joints or bends, becoming more porous and developing holes. Food molecules can leach through these

holes and enter the bloodstream. The food toxins in your bloodstream set off your natural alarm system. A few undigested food molecules don't cause a huge problem – your liver is called into action to deal with the toxins. But if the gut is very porous, the liver is quickly overrun and then these foreign bodies absorb into tissues throughout the body, causing them to inflame.

What causes a leaky gut?

Inflammation in the gut lining causes the microvilli filters that act as the barrier between our gut and our bloodstream to be swallowed up. The microvilli are like very fine hairs that protect the delicate gut wall from bigger undigested food molecules. If part of the microvilli are aggravated and inflamed, then those food molecules can get through the lining and become a toxin in the bloodstream.

This can be caused by:

A. **Diet:** refined sugars, processed foods, preservatives and refined flours. Too many toxins in the gut over many years means that the gut becomes inflamed as it just can't keep up.
B. **Stress:** stress almost always results in a suppressed immune system. A weakened immune system cannot handle doing its normal job and gets overrun more quickly, causing inflammation.
C. **Bad bacteria:** if the bacterial balance in your gut is wrong, the 'bad' bacteria can take over and lead to inflammation.

How do you know if you have a leaky gut?

Instead of or as well as gut-health problems (stomach cramps, bloating, diarrhoea) you may get:

- Multiple food sensitivities
- Frequent colds and illnesses
- Skin complaints such as eczema and rashes
- Headaches, brain fog and fatigue

THE BOTTOM LINE

Your gut-health problems, aches and pains and food intolerances could all be intrinsically linked. Let's start at the root of the problem, your gut, and see if we can understand it better. If we understand it and acquire the tools to fix it, then we can control and reduce the other symptoms too.

This 28-day plan is just the start. If you've been eating processed foods, refined flours and excessive sugar for twenty, thirty or forty plus years, then we can't fix the gut in one go. But we can take some huge, positive steps in the right direction and get you feeling better right now.

HOW TO IMPROVE YOUR GUT HEALTH

The 28-Day Gut-Health Plan is unique in its aim to dramatically improve the state of your gut in just 28 days. How does it do this? There are three practical and effective ways in which we tackle the health of your gut.

3 STEPS TO BETTER GUT HEALTH

1. Resting your gut

'Like a detox but with food.'

The Gut-Health Plan is not about starving yourself and eating less food. You will eat less, but this will be because of changes in your gut that will result in a reduction in cravings and choosing foods which will keep you fuller for longer. For the first week of the plan, called the Rest and Restore phase, you will remove the five most common trigger foods for a sensitive digestion. These foods are harder for your body to digest, so stay in your gut for longer, causing problems along the way.

The foods that you will eat in the Rest and Restore phase may seem quite restrictive, but you will notice an improvement relatively quickly. Essentially, by sticking to easily digested foods for at least a week, your digestive system doesn't need to work anywhere near as hard. It's a relaxing time for your digestion and it will reduce digestive stress. If the gut is not constantly working to digest food, it starts to recover and rebuild. This is a simple yet crucial part in the jigsaw of good gut health.

2. Reducing inflammation

Certain foods can cause the gut wall to react in a negative way. It can make the gut lining swollen, inflamed and extra sensitive. Now, the food triggers that cause inflammation are different for each person. But if we cut out ALL the common triggers during the Rest and Restore phase, then your gut lining has the best chance of getting back to normal. The gut cannot heal when it is inflamed.

3. Introducing good bacteria

The third crucial phase is to improve the balance of bacteria in our gut. We do this more quickly by adding probiotics to our diet for the duration of the programme. Of course, following the programme and reducing processed foods and wheat will slowly improve the bacterial balance anyway, but we are going to give it a helping hand. The best probiotics contain several different strains of bacteria as well as a high concentration of them. Improving bacterial balance means that the food you eat is better digested, which is important for gut health.

THE POWER OF GOOD BACTERIA

Your gut is chock-full of bacteria, good and bad. We can supplement our diet with probiotics (good bacteria) to help reverse the damage caused by years of junk-food overload. Probiotics are found naturally in some foods, particularly yogurt. But to really have an impact on our digestive systems, a probiotic supplement is the best way to ensure we have enough good bacteria to balance the gut effectively.

The good bacteria in a probiotic supplement will:

- Aid the digestion of complex foods and/or foods which you cannot currently digest
- Compete for space and nutrition with harmful bacteria, reducing their numbers and reducing stomach complaints
- Prevent toxins moving from the gut into the blood

Unfortunately, the popular probiotic drinks and enhanced foods don't really cut the mustard when it comes to supplementing. To get any real benefit, you need a probiotic tablet or powder. The number of different bacterial strains, together with the concentration of bacteria, is most important for success.

The most proven and the one now being prescribed by specialists for IBS and similar illnesses is a brand of probiotic called VSL3 (www.vsl3.co.uk). This brand contains the most strains of good bacteria and has 450 billion bacteria per sachet. But it is expensive and needs to be kept refrigerated.

THE BLOATING PROBLEM

Probiotics plus more fibre can lead to extra bloating in the first week of the programme. When you start taking probiotics you could get more bloated not less. But if you care about improving your gut health, it's a really important step. And in a strange way, it shows that the probiotics have started to do their job. They've started the battle and are breaking down foods that your body normally doesn't digest, producing more gas. Give the probiotics a week during the Rest and Restore phase and you'll see the bloating reduce. At the end of the week, your waist size and bloating will have reduced and be back to normal. You might even have lost weight and an inch or two round your tummy.

The more traumatized your gut the worse this will be. Give it a week. It will get better. And it means that a change for the better has begun. Don't start the Introducing phases until it is resolved.

FIBRE VS INTOLERANCE

One of the key tenets of improving your gut health and soothing your bowel symptoms is keeping levels of both soluble and insoluble fibre high. But look at this list of fibre-rich foods:

- Vegetables: broccoli (raw), cabbage, carrots (raw), peas and spinach
- Grains: whole grain-breads, whole-grain cereals, oatmeal and bran
- Beans/pulses: kidney beans, lima beans, black beans and lentils

And if we compare it with our list of top five food intolerances (see page 9), there's a huge overlap! Broccoli and cabbage are gassy vegetables, bread and cereals all contain wheat, and don't even get me started on how gassy beans can make you!

On the one hand, we need to restrict these possibly gut-intolerant foods. On the other, fibrous foods are needed to ensure smooth running of your insides. It's a real conundrum and one that we can only fully address when we reach the end of the 28-day plan.

During the programme, you should up your consumption of safe fibre-rich foods. Most fruits, especially bananas and berries, are safe and rich in fibre. Oats are particularly good as they are very easy for the body to digest and are an excellent source of fibre.

If you look at the recipes, I use the odd-sounding psyllium husks in various recipes including my Seeded Gluten-free Bread (see page 145). Psyllium is a powder that forms a fibrous gel on contact with water. It should be used sparingly but is perhaps one of the purest sources of fibre. It can be sprinkled onto breakfast cereal and added to recipes to improve fibre content.

Finally, buckwheat, which contrary to its name contains no wheat or gluten at all, is a fabulous source of fibre. I particularly like using buckwheat pasta as that opens up the way to lots of delicious pasta sauces and bakes.

If you suffer from either constipation or diarrhoea, then increasing the fibre in your diet (from non-problematic sources) can make stools softer (good for constipation) or bulkier and more regular (good for diarrhoea).

Be aware, though, that just like the addition of probiotics to your diet, increasing your fibre intake can initially lead to bloating and constipation. So if you are adding all of these at once at the start of the 28-day programme, then you may find that some symptoms, particularly bloating, increase during this time. If it becomes too uncomfortable, cut out the additional fibre and concentrate on the probiotics in the first instance. Fibre can be added gradually later when you have a better understanding of your food intolerances.

UNDERSTANDING YOUR OWN SENSITIVITIES

The 28-Day Gut-Health Plan is all about understanding your own sensitivities. We all react differently to different foods, and as so many factors influence our gut health it's often hard to pinpoint what's wrong and why.

Is it the slice of toast that gave you stomach cramps? Or nervousness about an exam? Perhaps it's your period? Or even the menopause? Did you sleep well last night?

By following this plan we are trying to cut out as many uncertainties as we can. We do this by eliminating the five most common food intolerances for a week. Then introduce the possible trigger foods one at a time. Key to success is accurate recording of symptoms using the **Gut-Health Diary** (see pages 97–128).

HOW MUCH WEIGHT CAN I LOSE?

The amazing bonus of the 28-Day Gut-Health Plan is the weight loss that goes hand in hand with improving your gut-health. This happens simply because you are cutting back on processed foods and sugars, eating foods that your body can digest and eating three filling and balanced meals a day.

When you first give up all trigger foods during the Rest and Restore week, the weight loss can be quite dramatic. As much as one pound a day in the first week. The rate of weight loss is obviously dependent on how much weight you have to lose, but you should expect upwards of three pounds in the first week. After this, the weight loss will settle down but you should continue to lose weight at a rate of one to three pounds a week, depending on your personal intolerances. This diet is not a 'fad' diet; it's a healthy way of eating and the weight loss is real and permanent.

TOP 5 WAYS TO MINIMIZE GUT STRESS

1. Don't eat big fatty meals

Make your meals smaller by reducing your plate size. Realize that a 'blow-out' meal like a takeaway, fish and chips or lots of red meat will antagonize the strongest gut. This is made worse if the meal is eaten late in the evening, as you 'sleep on your food'. Steer clear if you can. But if you can't, take probiotics for at least a week afterwards and consider trigger food elimination to reset the gut.

2. Keep alcohol and caffeine levels low

Sadly for those of us that love both coffee and wine, alcohol and caffeine can have a negative effect on the gut. Caffeine is a stimulant and makes the gut overactive and increases bowel movements. Alcohol irritates the gastrointestinal tract, so can make your symptoms worse. Additionally, both alcohol and caffeine make you more dehydrated. The good news is that it is rare to be intolerant to alcohol or caffeine, so neither needs to be eliminated entirely. Just be aware of their effects and try and reduce consumption during the programme and when your gut health is poor.

3. Drink more water

Increasing the amount of water you drink is perhaps the easiest way to improve your overall gut health. It simply helps keep everything within the gut moving smoothly. Always keep a water bottle to hand and make sure you drink whenever you are thirsty. Additionally, drink a glass of water first thing in the morning (to wake up your digestion) and make sure you drink at least one glass of water before every meal and more during the summer months.

Remember, caffeinated drinks are diuretic (make you more dehydrated) and the bubbles in carbonated drinks can pass through the body undigested and cause uncomfortable wind.

Short answer: Water is best!

4. Keep away from artificial sweeteners

Artificial sweeteners such as sorbitol and sucralose can cause diarrhoea and flatulence even if you have a healthy gut. All sweeteners that end with an -ol should be avoided and watch out for the use of different names on packaging that are meant to confuse you into thinking these sweeteners are natural. All sweeteners are considered toxins by the body and your gut tries to expel them quickly.

5. Avoid ready meals and shop-bought baked goods

Ready meals and shop-bought baked goods can contain hidden triggers, and even a small amount of a trigger food could set you back. Use the tips and recipes in the book to make simple real food quickly. Low-fat or reduced-calorie foods are particularly bad as the good bits have been sucked out along with the calories and replaced with empty and unnatural fillers that can irritate the gut lining.

INITIAL GUT ASSESSMENT QUIZ

This initial assessment is vital in getting a baseline reading of the state of your gut health. It will help you compare objectively to others. Importantly, it will help you to answer the question:

'Is it really that bad?'

YOUR OVERALL HEALTH

1. Do you have low energy or feel overly fatigued?

0	1	2	3	4	5	6	7	8	9	10

0 Never   10 Always

2. Do you consider yourself to be overweight?

0	1	2	3	4	5

0 Perfect Weight   2 A little bit overweight   4 Very overweight   5 Obese

3. Do you suspect you have food intolerances or allergies?

0	1	2	3	4	5	6	7	8	9	10

0 No   10 Strongly Suspect

INFLAMMATION

4. Do you have skin complaints? For example, itchy skin, rashes, eczema, rosacea, acne, hives, psoriasis.

0	1	2	3	4	5	6	7	8	9	10

0 No   5 Occasional   10 Yes, moderate to severe and/or multiple

5. Do you have hay fever, dust or pet allergies?

0	1	2	3	4	5	6	7	8	9	10

0 No   5 Some, unmedicated   10 Yes, medicated and severe

6. Do you experience joint pain or unexplained muscle pain?

0	1	2	3	4	5

0 Never   3 A little   5 Daily

7. Do you suffer from frequent sinus pain or other sinus-related issues?

0	1	2	3	4	5

0 No   2 Occasionally   5 Yes, often

8. Do you get problems such as brain fog, chronic headaches, anxiety?

0	1	2	3	4	5	6	7	8	9	10

0 Never   5 Occasionally   10 Yes, often

YOUR DIGESTION

On average, and when eating without restrictions, how many **days a week** do you suffer from:

9. Stomach cramps:

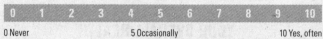

0	1	2	3	4	5	6	7

10. Diarrhoea:

0	1	2	3	4	5	6	7

11. Constipation:

| 0 | 1 | 2 | 3 | 4 | 5 | 6 | 7 |

12. Bloating:

| 0 | 1 | 2 | 3 | 4 | 5 | 6 | 7 |

13. Acid reflux:

| 0 | 1 | 2 | 3 | 4 | 5 | 6 | 7 |

14. Excessive wind:

| 0 | 1 | 2 | 3 | 4 | 5 | 6 | 7 |

WORKING OUT YOUR SCORE

Add up the scores for every question (1–14) and use the chart below to check the current state of your gut health.

Gut-Health Total..

Total Points	Gut-Health Score
9 or below	1
10–14	2
15–19	3
20–24	4
25–34	5
35–39	6
40–44	7
45–54	8
55–59	9
60 or above	10

My Gut-Health Score...

WHAT DOES YOUR GUT-HEALTH SCORE MEAN?

9–10 Severe

Disrupts your everyday life.

You may already be under the care of your doctor, and if not you should consider it.

The Gut-Health Plan may help you but you should also take medical advice. Be prepared for the programme to take longer than normal, and to find many food sensitivities.

7–8 Moderate to Severe

Although your gut health doesn't bother you every day, you suffer more often than not and are always thinking about it.

The Gut-Health Plan should help you to get to grips with your gut-health. You are likely to find one or more food sensitivity.

3–6 Mild to Moderate

Your gut health doesn't affect you every day. But it is slowly but surely getting worse. You might find that it gets worse during periods of stress and uncertainty and at inconvenient times, such as when you are on holiday.

The good news is that this programme can help reverse the flow and help you understand and improve your gut health.

1–2 Mild

You may suffer from occasional symptoms. You are unlikely to have any intolerances. If you feel that your gut health is getting worse, then this programme will get you back to optimum gut health.

THE 5 BIG TRIGGERS

During the 28-Day Gut-Health Plan we are concentrating on the five most common food triggers for gut health:

1. Lactose (Milk)
2. Red Meat
3. Nightshade family (tomatoes, (bell) peppers, chilli peppers, aubergine)
4. Gas-producing (gassy) Vegetables (onions, garlic, broccoli, beans)
5. Wheat

We are concentrating here on **food intolerances** as opposed to **allergies**.

An intolerance:

- Develops over time
- Gets worse as you get older
- Doesn't always affect you in the same way
- Can allow you to still eat the food in smaller quantities

With food allergies, you are either born with them or develop them as a young child. The reaction to foods is intense with only a very small quantity. Your food allergy may have involved medical treatment of some kind, although there is no cure. If you have an allergy, it is very black and white. You know about it and are hopefully receiving medical support. For our purposes, being coeliac is definitely an allergy. If you have an allergy, you can still find support for other possible food intolerances in this book and hopefully find recipes that support your allergy and your lifestyle.

Remember that any food intolerances develop from an underlying gut-health problem. You can inherit gut-health problems or they can be caused by the foods you eat and the lifestyle you follow. This is why gut-health symptoms tend to worsen as you get older.

We start to mend the gut by first introducing probiotics. These will improve the bacterial balance. Foods will be digested better and are less likely to come into contact with the gut wall. Although probiotics will improve your entire gut, it is a slow process and doesn't deal directly with any food intolerances you might have developed.

For this reason, in addition to the probiotics, we start the 28-Day Plan with a 7-Day Rest and Restore phase that removes the five common food triggers from your diet. By removing the intolerance (the food that your body considers most toxic), we can reduce the inflammation in the lining of the gut. It is only then that the gut can start to heal.

When the gut has started to heal and symptoms have reduced, we can then reintroduce trigger foods gradually and see what effects they have on YOUR body. The aim of the programme is not only to improve the health of your gut, but also to understand your own specific food intolerances so that you can learn to balance the foods you eat with the effect they have on your body.

We introduce food groups in a particular order, with the trickiest and most difficult triggers to diagnose coming last – gassy vegetables and wheat.

LACTOSE (MILK)

Lactose or milk sugar is a sugar found only in milk or milk products.

Milk vs Dairy

A common misconception, however, is that anything made from milk contains lactose. Which is why some people may be confused and eliminate all dairy from their diet.

Dairy does define all food made from milk. However, in 'hard' or solid dairy products such as butter or cheese all the lactose has been removed. If you think back to domestic science, or perhaps even the nursery rhyme, milk is split into curds and whey. Curds is the solid protein and fat and contains no lactose.

An even simpler definition is:

'If you have to cut it with a knife, it's safe.'

Milk (lactose) foods to avoid

Milk, all types including skimmed and semi-skimmed

Cream

Custard

Fromage frais

Ghee

Ice cream

Margarine

Sour cream

Yogurt

Milk or white chocolate

Soft cheese such as cottage cheese, cream cheese, halloumi

Additionally, check the ingredients list on: cereals, baked goods, crisps, cooked meats and soups. Look out for any of these in the nutritional information, as they all signify lactose: casein, caseinates, sodium caseinates, hydrolysed casein, milk powder, milk solids.

Safe dairy foods

Butter

Hard cheese such as Cheddar, feta and Parmesan

Note that eggs are not a dairy food, contain no lactose and can be eaten safely.

Using lactose-free milk to simplify the removal of milk lactose from your diet

Lactose-free milk is now commonly available in every supermarket and is a really simple way to cut out lactose from your diet and see if it makes a difference to your gut health. You can also buy lactose-free yogurts, soft cheese and cream.

RED MEAT

Red meat can be problematic for your gut health for two reasons:

1. Red meat is simply one of the hardest things for your gut to break down and digest. It is often the case that occasional small quantities of red meat are OK for all but the most sensitive digestions. But increase the quantities, eat it late at night or together with a large, fatty meal and the likelihood of a problem increases hugely.

2. The other problem with red meat can be bacterial. This could mean that you have a problem with one meat in particular, be that beef, pork or lamb. This sometimes happens if you've had a bad bout of meat-related food poisoning in the past. The gut becomes colonized by the bad bacteria and you stay sensitive for years afterwards. Probiotics really help here as they can reduce or eliminate the problematic bacteria.

On the plus side, it is unlikely that you will have to eliminate red meat entirely from your diet. Just remember moderation is always the key to avoiding problems with red meat. If you do have a problem, cut out all red meat for at least forty-eight hours until all symptoms have passed.

Red meat to avoid

All forms of beef, lamb, pork and game	Duck
Minced beef	Game
Burgers	Bacon
Sausages	Salami
Ham	Chorizo

White meat (you can eat as much as you like)

Chicken

Turkey

All parts of the bird can be eaten, including the dark meat, such as turkey thigh.

NIGHTSHADE

Fruits from the nightshade family – tomatoes, bell peppers, chillies and aubergines (eggplants) – contain glycoalkaloids and/or capsaicin, which are surprisingly common triggers for a sensitive gut. It is estimated that as many as one in three of us could be sensitive to nightshades, although for many people it is a minor rather than major intolerance.

The highest concentration of glycoalkaloids is found in tomatoes. Tomatoes, either fresh, tinned or in pastes or passatas, are harder to avoid than you might imagine. Many dishes, from stews to curries, have tomatoes as their base. The problem with glycoalkaloids is that they can destroy cell membranes and can 'burst open' cells. This property is part of their natural defence against small mammals and birds that like to eat the sweet fruits of these plants. To the smaller stomachs of these animals, the glycoalkaloids have a toxic effect. As a much bigger animal, humans should be immune to their effects, but unfortunately, weakened gut linings have made people more susceptible to their effects. It has been suggested that by damaging the gut lining they may be one of the causes of leaky gut.

The other molecule in these red (and green) fruits is the tricky capsaicin. Capsaicin has a very different but equally nasty effect on the gut. Capsaicin is an irritant, and in the same way that you get pain and watery eyes if you just touch your eyes after chopping a chilli, capsaicin can irritate and inflame the gut lining, causing stomach cramps and pain. All chillies, fresh, dried or in powder form, contain the dreaded capsaicin. In fact, all red spices – e.g. paprika, chilli powder, cayenne pepper – contain concentrated capsaicin and should be avoided.

Fresh chilli peppers contain both glycoalkaloids and capsaicin, so are 'the perfect storm' when it comes to nightshade sensitivity.

Foods to avoid

Fresh tomatoes	Chilli paste
Tinned tomatoes	Chilli sauce
Tomato purée	Jalapeños
Tomato ketchup	Paprika
Peppers (bell) – red, green, yellow and orange	Mild or hot chilli powder
	Curry powder
Aubergine (eggplant)	Madras powder
Chilli peppers	Cayenne pepper
Pimento peppers	

Basically the food rule is:

'Steer clear of red foods.'

GAS-PRODUCING (GASSY) VEGETABLES

Most of the carbohydrate foods we eat release bubbles of gas as they are digested. In some people, it is not the gas in itself that causes the problem; it is how our bodies deal with the bubbles. If you are sensitive to gas-producing foods then it is likely that you suffer from painful stomach cramps as the gas gets trapped and your body tries to push it through the digestive tract. Unfortunately this gets worse at night as we are lying down 'at rest' and the natural movement of the body and gravity are not there to help push the gas away.

Gas-producing vegetables are perhaps the most common problem for people with a sensitive gut. Some troublesome veggies such as beans and cauliflower are relatively easy to avoid. But perhaps the most difficult foods are onions and garlic. They are incredibly tricky to steer clear of because they make their way into all sorts of unexpected foodstuffs, being a key flavouring for many meals. And secondly, they are the absolute worst at causing the production of gas. Even a tiny amount can trigger a reaction and cause a sleepless night.

Total abstinence from these foods is advised. I know this is difficult, but it might just be the root of so many gut issues that it is absolutely worth the effort. Use the recipes in this book to help. There is a huge variety of meals and flavours to stop your food being bland. Then learn the few key food swaps – lactose-free milk, celery, asafoetida and garlic oil (see pages 51–2) – that can really make things easier. And think positive … You may never have to chop an onion again!

Foods to avoid
Onions and garlic

Red onion	Garlic
White onion	Garlic paste
Spring (green) onion (white part)	Garlic flavouring
Onion powder	Garlic salt
Onion flavouring	Leeks

Note that the green part of a spring onion is allowed, as are chives and celery. Garlic oil is also allowed (and makes a fantastic substitute). The damaging part of the garlic is not soluble in oil, so a garlic-infused oil contains lots of garlic flavour without any of the risks.

Other vegetables

Broccoli	Kale
Cauliflower	Cabbage

Beans and lentils

All kinds of beans including:

Kidney beans	Borlotti beans
Baked beans	Black-eyed beans
Haricot (navy) beans	Soy beans
Butter beans (lima beans)	

All kinds of lentils including:

Red lentils
Brown lentils
Puy lentils

Chickpeas should also be avoided.

WHEAT

If you have a fat tummy, love handles or 'man boobs', you are not alone. Look around you. The characteristic paunch is extremely common. It gets worse as you get older, and is virtually impossible to shift through diet and exercise. What if this unshiftable belly is caused by twenty years of wheat overload? There's new thinking that suggests that wheat could be the primary cause of your inflated belly and bloating.

Why avoid wheat?

Not all carbs are the same. Starchy or complex carbs such as rice, oats and potatoes release their energy more slowly than sugar, which is a simple carbohydrate. But isn't wheat a complex carbohydrate? Yes. But it has unique properties that actually make it release its energy at the same rate as sugar.

Think about how much wheat you eat daily. It's probably part of every meal. And if you have a snack it's likely to be present there too. Could the problem be wheat overload? We know that wheat cannot be fully digested and may cause small tears to appear in the intestines.

Cut out wheat entirely

As wheat is in so much of the food you eat you'll need to start looking at the packaging of every food you buy. Even better, stick to whole, natural foods which don't come in a packet, and get back to basics with your cooking.

Foods to avoid

Bread	Malt or malt extract
Cake	Pasta
Biscuits	Noodles
Pastries	Pancakes
Pies	Breakfast cereals
Crackers	Barley
Pitta or wraps	Rye
Beer	Bulgur wheat

Gluten-free products – good or bad?

You need to approach gluten-free food products with caution. These processed foods are often full of very quick-release carbohydrates such as rice flour and sugar. Your best bet is to prepare your own food, which you can guarantee as gluten-free naturally.

However, I have found that it helps to feel less restricted if you can have access to a gluten-free bread now and again. We are lucky that there are now hundreds of gluten-free products available. If you find a gluten-free bread that you like, then you should treat yourself occasionally. Even better, buy a gluten-free bread flour and make your own gluten-free bread. I have perfected my own recipe for this and you'll find it in the **Step Up Recipes** section.

EVERYBODY IS DIFFERENT

MY OWN JOURNEY

- Jacqueline, in her forties
- Symptoms – bloating

I used to feel bloated even after eating a small meal. Bloating is so subjective, it's hard to know the exact cause and solution. I didn't tend to feel poorly, so it was hard to pin it down to any one cause. I also got eczema on my face and had a tendency to migraines.

After much experimentation last year (this programme is intended to cut out the grey areas allowing you to reach your own conclusions much quicker), I discovered that wheat was the problem. The difficulty is that with bloating caused by wheat intolerance (which is so common), it doesn't come straight after eating wheat; it comes maybe a day later and lasts about forty-eight hours. So if I eat wheat on the Monday, I might not get symptoms until Tuesday and they won't completely disappear until Thursday. It's so easy to eat a little bit of wheat every day and then the bloating never really goes away.

I cut out wheat completely for a few months and felt a lot better for it. My eczema cleared up nicely and the frequency of my migraines decreased. All due to cutting out wheat.

That's not quite the end of the story. And this may be familiar to some of you. I was feeling better and I knew this was due to cutting out wheat. I wanted to try and reintroduce it slowly. I missed bread. And the first few times I experimented with bread it seemed fine. A bit of bloating the day after eating wheat is easy to overlook. Unfortunately, this led to me, almost imperceptibly, going back to eating wheat every day. And slowly but surely my symptoms returned. It took seeing my stomach in the mirror to acknowledge it. My tummy was not fatty or flabby ... just bloated.

My new plan, which I have been following successfully for the past few months, is to cut out wheat entirely once again. But I make a wheat-free loaf of bread and eat gluten-free bread most days (see page 145). I have to use a rice flour to make the bread, which isn't ideal. But I have realized that total wheat restriction is no fun in the long run. So my long-term rules for me are: no wheat and no processed foods. But if I want to eat chocolate, gluten-free bread or make some cookies containing real sugar, I do.

Let's hear from some other people I have helped find their own trigger foods, and who enjoy their life more due to a greater understanding of their gut health.

ANGELA

- Angela, in her fifties
- Symptoms – stomach cramps at night

Angela has been getting stomach cramps at night for thirty years. Not every night, but sometimes they are so bad that she barely sleeps at all. She noticed a correlation with nightshade, so for a long time she has avoided tomatoes in all their forms. Her symptoms became progressively worse over the years. She then tried removing wheat and dairy from her diet with little success.

It was only on total removal of all gas-producing foods that her symptoms improved.

Angela's triggers are nightshade and gas-producing vege-tables. In particular, she knows that even a tiny bit of onion or garlic will trigger her symptoms. Tomatoes in small doses and cooked tinned tomatoes are less of a problem.

Her solution is to avoid onions, garlic, leeks, beans and lentils totally. She also takes probiotics when her stomach is weak or when she needs antibiotics. She takes a fibre supple-ment (a teaspoon of ground psyllium) daily.

Angela allows herself to consume tomatoes and peppers in small amounts up to three times a week. She also eats wheat and dairy freely.

STEPHEN

- Stephen, in his forties
- Symptoms – loose bowels

Stephen is a busy executive who has a stressful job. In a particularly difficult period at work, his symptoms became unbearable and made it difficult for him to do his job properly.

On the advice of the doctor, he cut out all five triggers until his symptoms abated. Then, after a long period of trial and error, it became clear that it was the milk in his many cups of tea that was the problem. Stress also exacerbated the symptoms. His treatment involved probiotics for three weeks to rebuild the gut.

He now does not have milk or yogurt, although cheese is fine. He also is careful about how much red meat he eats. Meat in moderation is fine, but overindulgence can cause his symptoms to reappear.

ANTONIA

- Antonia, in her thirties
- Symptoms – severe stomach cramps, bloating

Antonia found her symptoms were making her miserable and interfering with her life. She chose to take a food-intolerance test, which highlighted red meat, milk and wheat.

Antonia avoids these three triggers entirely and she is now symptom-free.

JOHN

- John, in his seventies
- Symptoms – bloating

John didn't feel he had any intolerances or symptoms. However, he did notice that he was bloated after meals and struggled to lose weight despite eating more healthily. John consumed a lot of wheat (as many of us do), so he decided to cut it out for one month to see if he noticed the difference. After a month wheat-free he felt so much better – more energy, no bloating and yes ... he'd lost half a stone.

John now eats wheat only on special occasions – a rustic roll in a restaurant or a piece of homemade birthday cake – with no symptoms, but he knows that if he eats wheat more regularly his symptoms will return.

FOOD AND DRINK

You may be wondering what on earth you can safely eat on the programme. There's plenty of truly nutritious and safe food that's available and not too complicated to make. I'll also introduce you to some great **Healing Foods** (that can help your gut recover faster) and some **Hero Foods** that add lots of flavour without risking your gut.

SAFE FOODS

These are the foods that you know are 100 per cent safe to eat at any stage of the plan.

Meat, fish and eggs

Chicken	Prawns
Turkey	Salmon
Eggs	Tuna
Fish	Tofu

Dairy and alternatives

Lactose-free milk	Feta
Almond milk	Brie
Soya milk	Goat's cheese
Coconut milk	Mozzarella
Butter	Swiss cheese
Cheddar	Parmesan

Vegetables

Carrot	Fennel
Bean sprouts	Ginger
Green beans	Lettuce
Beetroot	Rocket (arugula)
Pak choi	Peas
Celery	Potatoes (without skin)
Celeriac	Spinach
Chives	Sweet potato
Spring onion (green part only)	Butternut squash
Sweetcorn	Swiss chard
Courgette	Water chestnuts
Cucumber	

Fruit

Avocado	Kiwi
Banana	Melon
Blueberries	Pineapple
Orange	Pomegranate seeds
Satsuma/clementine	Raspberries
Lemon	Strawberries
Lime	Rhubarb
Grapes	

Nuts and seeds

Almonds (ground almonds)

Walnuts

Hazelnuts

Macadamia nuts

Peanuts

Pecans

Pine nuts

Chia seeds

Pumpkin seeds

Sesame seeds

Sunflower seeds

Grains and cereals

Oats

Rice

Buckwheat

Cornflour (cornstarch)

Oatbran

Polenta

Quinoa

Fats and Oils

Mild olive oil

Olive oil

Extra-virgin olive oil

Confectionery and sugar

Dark chocolate

Honey

White sugar

Brown sugar

Maple syrup

Herbs and spices

Basil	Thyme
Chives	Cinnamon
Coriander (cilantro)	Cumin
Ginger	Five spice
Parsley	Star anise
Rosemary	Turmeric
Tarragon	Asafoetida

Sauces

Mustard	Peanut butter
Tamari (wheat-free) soy sauce	Mirin
Maple syrup	Worcestershire sauce
Balsamic vinegar	Fish sauce
Apple cider vinegar	

HEALING FOODS

If you want foods that not only are 'safe' but also help heal the gut from the inside then these are my absolute top foods. Some, like kombucha, help reduce inflammation of the gut, some improve the bacterial balance and others help the digestive tract run more smoothly.

Apple cider vinegar and balsamic vinegar

Both these vinegars taste amazing and are so versatile. I make a simple salad dressing with both and it is absolutely delicious. Apple cider vinegar and authentic balsamic are fermented foods. Fermented foods are natural sources of really good gut bacteria. These bacteria complement those found in probiotics and help you gain the best balance. Both vinegars also contain acetic acid (it's what makes them sharp) which helps lower the sugar that we absorb from our food. Here is my perfect go-to salad dressing …

Everyday Healing Vinaigrette

> Simply mix together 1 tbsp extra-virgin olive oil, 2 tsp apple cider vinegar, ½ tsp balsamic vinegar, ½ tsp English mustard and a generous seasoning of salt and black pepper.

Kombucha

Kombucha is a fermented tea drink. It naturally inhibits the growth of harmful bacteria and has a soothing and anti-inflammatory effect on the gut lining. If you think you have a leaky gut and it is making inflammatory conditions such as arthritis and acne worse, then kombucha may be beneficial for you. There are some amazing online shops selling kombucha drinks that are worth hunting down. And if you find the drink helpful, you can then go on to make your own easily and relatively inexpensively.

Tamari wheat-free soy sauce

Instead of standard soy sauce, you can now buy tamari soy sauce from most supermarkets. It's a fraction more expensive but not disastrously so. Naturally fermented and wheat-free, it adds different bacterial strains to the probiotic mix.

Psyllium husks

Psyllium is a prebiotic powder that you can buy from health-food shops. I recommend it as it's the purest and simplest way of adding prebiotics to your diet. Prebiotics are a special type of fibre that complement probiotics as they encourage the growth of good bacteria in your gut. Think of prebiotics as food for the good bacteria. Once you have 'sown the seed' of probiotics, prebiotics will encourage the good bacteria to grow and flourish. Additionally, the fibre element helps keep your digestive system running smoothly and relieves both diarrhoea and constipation symptoms.

I use psyllium in gluten-free bread recipes, but you can also dissolve a teaspoon in water or juice. It is a very concentrated fibre source, so it is important to drink at least two glasses of water or juice with every teaspoon.

Olive oil

The more natural the oil or fat the better. For this reason the ONLY fats I use in cooking are olive oil and butter. Olive oil is by far the least processed of the oils we use and has a very high percentage of heart-healthy monounsaturated fat. You can get olive oil in three varieties (and I use them all): 'normal' olive oil is my go-to oil for frying and general cooking, extra-virgin olive oil is fabulous in salad dressings and mild (or light) olive oil is great for baking or anywhere you just need an oil without the olive oil flavour.

HERO FOODS

When you're avoiding whole food groups, it's easy to feel that you're cutting out all the flavour and excitement from your food. After all, if you cut out meat, tomatoes, onion and wheat, what is left?

Actually, there is plenty, but to avoid bland food you have to be a little bit clever with your food swaps. You'll find that I use all of the swaps listed here in the Gut-Health Plan Recipes and they are key to moving forward and living with food intolerances, whether just for the short term or if you find you need to avoid these foods for the foreseeable future.

Lactose-free milk

Lactose-free milk can now be found in any supermarket; it's only a little bit more expensive than your standard semi-skimmed. What's more, you can't taste the difference, so it's one of the easiest swaps ever. There are also lactose-free yogurts and ice cream but they are a little bit harder to find.

Onions and garlic

Onions and garlic are perhaps the hardest foods to avoid. If you think about it, the vast majority of our meals contain them in some form or another. If you're buying pre-prepared food, it's practically guaranteed. The problem is exacerbated by the fact that only a small quantity can set off an intolerance, so we need to be very careful indeed.

Garlic oil

Garlic oil is extra-virgin olive oil infused with garlic. Unlike garlic powder or pastes, the oil picks up the flavour of the garlic but without the troublesome 'gassy' molecules. This is because the garlic is not soluble in the oil, but it is in water. Garlic oil is brilliant because it can be used in practically any dish that requires garlic. Simply substitute 1 teaspoon of garlic oil for 1 clove of crushed garlic. Garlic oil is completely safe for sensitive tummies. You could also try chilli oil as a great way to add heat to a dish without the chilli.

Celery

Celery should be your go-to onion substitute in many dishes. It has a slightly milder flavour than onion. But if you add one or two chopped celery sticks in the place of an onion in a dish, particularly a traditional British dish like Cottage Pie (see page 187), then you won't notice the difference.

Asafoetida

If you've not heard of asafoetida before, you are not alone. It's not a commonly used spice outside of the Indian sub-continent. A yellow spice, also called 'hing', it can be purchased cheaply and easily from the supermarket. In cooking it adds a mild onion or leek flavour to any dish. You need about a teaspoon as a substitute for an onion and it does add a yellow colour. It really is fantastic for adding warmth and depth of flavour to a dish. I'm a total convert and use it in many dishes.

THE PROBLEM WITH PROCESSED FOODS

Here's the thing: processed foods are bad for you. We all know it. But they are immensely hard to avoid. They are the primary cause of the modern obesity epidemic and the root cause of so many food allergies and intolerances. Honestly, I would prefer it if you ate a huge slice of homemade chocolate cake, rather than one 'healthy' shop-bought granola bar.

Processing brings preservatives, colourants and flavourings. But it also has no regard for the delicate balance of our gut. The refining and sanitizing of the product, together with hidden sugars and unnatural chemicals, means that any processed or pre-prepared meal is an alien invader on the sensitive gut.

How do we define a processed food?

As a simple rule of thumb:

> 'If it has an ingredients list and that
> list contains more than three ingredients,
> then that is a processed food.'

This isn't as bad as it sounds! Obviously meat, cheese, milk and vegetables are all fine as they don't have an ingredients list at all. And we are not ruling out food that has been tinned or processed for longer life, either. Tinned tomatoes, for example, are fine. As is smoked salmon. You've also got all those blessed timesavers like pre-cooked rice, ready-to-eat lentils or beans, or pasta. You can even have bread – as long as you make it yourself …

But we are getting ahead of ourselves. A lot of these foods need to be banished temporarily while we get on top of the current condition.

TIME FOR A REBOOT?

Think of the 28-Day Gut-Health Plan as a month of bed rest and recuperation for your gut. At the end of the programme, not only will your gut health have improved and your weight reduced, but other seemingly unrelated conditions such as migraines and eczema might also have cleared up.

> 'The 28-Day Programme cuts out some real food ... but only temporarily as a way of short-circuiting and rebooting the system.'

The ultimate goal of the plan is for you to be able to eat all the trigger foods in moderation, and the key to that is a life-long avoidance of processing. Yes, that means more cooking. And it means if you want a cake or a cookie, you'll have to make it yourself. But there are plenty of ways to prepare healthy food quickly. And through the recipes and guidance here you'll find speedy and simple ways to make real food from scratch in minutes.

DENIAL VS BALANCE

Some digestive issues come from an overindulgence in foods like wheat and dairy over time. You may need to deny yourself these foods during the plan because of many years of overindulgence. But when the plan has finished you should know much more about your trigger foods and how to avoid them. Foods that you thought were a problem might not be a trigger at all. And the majority of people find that their trigger foods can be incorporated on occasion with no ill effects.

Moderation is the key. A really big meal containing lots of your trigger foods or one which is exceptionally fatty or calorific might well trigger a problem.

'Your gut is a sensitive soul who can easily take offence. Treat it nicely and it will reward you by behaving sensibly for many years to come.'

FOOD AND DRINK FAQS

Can I drink beer?

For some people, the thought of giving up beer is rather terrifying. The commonly seen beer belly is one and the same as the dreaded 'wheat tummy'. Beer and lager contain gluten and need to be cut out for the duration of the programme. It could, however, be used as the test food in the Introducing ... Wheat and Gluten phase (see page 215).

Wine and spirits?

The good news is that wine and spirits are allowed in moderation. Red wine has a positive effect on the metabolism, as it contains antioxidants and other natural anti-inflammatories. Alcohol is digested by the body in a similar fashion to sugar, which is why we need to limit our consumption for weight-loss purposes. Don't drink too much in one night as you will get food cravings and your chances of accidentally eating a trigger food are much increased.

What about fizzy or carbonated drinks?

Try to avoid all fizzy or sparkling drinks as this directly introduces bubbles of gas into the gut. This gas can get trapped if your gut is not working efficiently and could cause stomach cramps.

Should I add sweeteners to drinks?

If you have a sensitive gut, then all sweeteners (and products containing sweeteners) should be avoided at all costs. The reason is simple. by their very nature, sweeteners are very poorly absorbed by the gut. They are not recognized as a foodstuff and your body will attempt to pass them out of the digestive system as quickly as possible. The result ... digestive system upheaval. If you crave something sweet, then have fruit or something with a small amount of real sugar in it. Sugar may be calorific but it is natural and very easily digested.

Can I drink tea, coffee and caffeine?

You may have heard that caffeinated drinks are bad for a sensitive gut. And yes, in an ideal world we would not include caffeine in this programme. Caffeine is a stimulant so may cause cramps and other symptoms to worsen. But it is not an irritant or inflammatory so will not make your gut symptoms worse on its own. I don't recommend removing caffeine from your diet as you start this programme, simply because it's too hard. You're giving up lots of things and changing your diet significantly. Cutting out caffeine suddenly results in additional food cravings and headaches.

If you don't drink caffeinated drinks, then great, but if you do, don't change your consumption at this stage. Of course, if you drink tea or coffee with milk, you'll have to swap to lactose-free for at least the first week of the plan.

How much water should I drink?

You can't have too much water. I know it's boring, but water is refreshing and good for you. You should aim to drink about eight glasses of water a day.

What about fruit teas?

A fruit tea, or a chamomile, peppermint or similar is just the ticket when you want something non-caffeinated and warming. There are so many to choose from these days, so stick to your favourite if you have one or try a selection if you are new to them.

RESTING YOUR STOMACH OVERNIGHT

An important part of this programme is allowing your digestive system time to rebuild and relax. The most obvious time for rest is during the night. If you still have food in your gut overnight, then this will jam up the system and not allow the body the valuable hours to rebuild. When you're awake and moving around, gravity and the motion of the body work in harmony helping the digestive system to work at the right speed. Overnight, your gut system attempts to shut down. But if there is still food in there, it just sits like a lump in your gut, weighing you down until morning.

As a rule of thumb, have your main meal at least three hours before you go to sleep, preferably four hours if you can manage it. Make sure you don't eat anything (although non-caffeinated hot or cold drinks are allowed) in the last ninety minutes before bed.

IS YOUR LIFESTYLE AFFECTING YOUR GUT?

Now you have all the pieces of the nutritional puzzle that make up a healthy gut, it is important to understand how other factors affect your body and your digestion.

Your hormones are strongly affected by environmental factors such as sleep, caffeine, alcohol, hydration and stress. If you don't consider these factors then you will not be getting the most from this plan. Although you may not appreciate it yet, your choices regarding these factors are just as important as your decisions related to the foods you eat.

If you've wondered why certain foods can affect you badly sometimes and not at other times, then you must look at the choices you make in these areas and make adjustments. It's not rocket science and if you want a truly healthy gut, as well as a healthier outlook on life, then you need to start here.

STRESS

Life is stressful. Everyone is different, but we all have some stress in our lives. What if we could turn down our stress and eliminate some or all of it from our lives? Yes, that's right, we'd be healthier and leaner too. Ever gone to bed worrying about a problem that seems insurmountable, but by morning it seems tiny and not worth the bother? It's called making a mountain out of a molehill and we do it all the time. There is stress we can control and stress we can't and it all takes its toll on our bodies.

It's clear that for many of us there is a direct link between being overstressed and a deterioration in our gut health. It is likely that the tension we feel when stressed can be a contributing factor to our digestive issues. The tension we can feel in our shoulders, neck and head, is also present in our gut. We don't experience the tension in our colon like we do in other parts of the body, but the tension can cause the normal regular contractions that push food through the gut to speed up and become stronger. Even with a healthy gut, we can still experience butterflies or cramps before an important event. When your gut is weakened in any way, small everyday stresses can have an impact, too. And if we have elevated stress levels for more than a short period of time, the gut is constantly tense and cannot operate normally.

We already have the tools to reduce our stress levels. But we need to be aware of when we are overstressed and make it our priority to deal with it before it starts to affect our mood or sleep patterns.

Have too much work on and find yourself working late into the night? Stop. Give yourself a time limit and definitely stop then. You will work faster and better the next day. Worrying about your children, a friend or an argument? If there's nothing you can do about it today, then make sure you switch off your thoughts along with your phone. Concentrate on something else – like a book or TV – and allow yourself to relax. When you think about it in the morning, it won't seem as bad and you may even have come up with the perfect solution in your dreams.

SLEEP

A good night's sleep improves your mood, burns fat and slows the ageing process. When you consider that, is it really important to stay up late watching rubbish telly? Or is it just a habit that has become the norm? If you consider yourself to be a night owl, then a good proportion of this is down to your own training and reinforcement of bad habits. Reset them slowly, by trying to go to bed five minutes earlier each night.

Eight full hours of sleep is what you need to aim for; any less than this and you will be more tempted by snacks, especially junk food and sweet treats, the next day. Also, in the later hours of the night, you'll start burning fat. If you only sleep for six hours you may not reach this zone and you'll still be burning last night's dinner!

Of course, an upset digestive system can disrupt your sleep considerably. This is why, when you've reset your system and started testing out your food intolerances, we try when possible to add these foods for the first time when you eat lunch. Although a food item can affect you for twenty-four to forty-eight hours after eating it, stomach cramps normally occur two to six hours after food.

Keeping track of your sleep and the interaction of your digestion and sleep patterns is key to understanding the impact of foods on your gut. Here are my 'sleep training' tips to getting quality sleep. You'll be amazed by the effect on your mood and your weight.

1. Start preparing for bed by 10 p.m. at the latest. That means: TV off, devices away, bright lights turned off or dimmed.
2. Relax. Ten–twenty minutes of your bedtime routine should be dedicated to some 'you time'. You could read a book, listen to the radio, put on your favourite music, have a bath, etc. The most important thing is to remove yourself from bright screens, get warm and cosy and turn off your brain.
3. Don't eat for at least two hours before bedtime. As I've already said, it's better for gut health to digest your food while you are still up and about and moving around. If you are going to have any problems with your stomach overnight, it will help to minimize it if the food has been sufficiently digested before bedtime.
4. Have a herbal drink. If you've got a hot herbal drink that you like, then warm and relax yourself with your favourite. Chamomile is good for sleep, but peppermint, rooibos or any fruity non-caffeinated drink is lovely and relaxing. About 9 p.m. is a good time to settle down with a cup of your favourite tea.

Finally, a quick word for those of you who look at this and laugh, thinking, 'Well for X or Y reason, eight hours' sleep is never gonna happen.' Maybe you've got babies, poorly children or have health problems that stop you getting a full night's sleep. For you a short nap in the afternoon will help enormously. Taking a thirty-minute power nap or a longer two-hour snooze will allow you to reset your hormone levels and control hunger and cravings. A nap doesn't make up for a good night's sleep but it is the next best thing.

HORMONAL CYCLE

Any woman reading this will know that their monthly cycle affects their gut in some way. Unfortunately, as it affects us all so differently, it's hard to make suggestions that will help everyone.

Let's start with what we do know. Your gut is most likely to be affected by your symptoms at the same time as you get other menstrual symptoms. So if you've got sore breasts and bloating, then you might notice an increase in your bowel movements as well. Although this varies from person to person, you are most likely to be suffering from these symptoms for a couple of days before the start of your period and for the first two to three days of your cycle.

Although there's not much we can do about a change in gut sensitivity due to the menstrual cycle, we can be aware of it and make adjustments and allowances. This means that if you are monitoring your gut health during your period you should note down where in your cycle you are and what effect, if any, your period might be having on your gut sensitivity. If you are in one of the phases of introducing new foods into your diet, be especially aware that your period might be making you score more highly for gut symptoms during the phase. If in any doubt, restart the Introducing ... recipes at the end of your period.

If you are at menopausal age or beyond, again the changes in your body can affect the gut. Your digestion is a very sensitive beast and doesn't like change. The hormonal changes that are taking place in your body are not set to any timescale. And just as this confuses your brain, it also confuses your gut. The nerve receptors in your gut are affected by a decrease in oestrogen in much the same way as they would be around your monthly period. The difference is that this doesn't follow a regular pattern as during your period, and symptoms can come more frequently and when you least expect them.

The only piece of good news on the horizon is that when you have gone through the menopause and come out the other side, your gut health should improve. By taking varying hormone levels out of the picture, there's one less disruptive signal for the gut to contend with.

EXERCISE

Never fear, I am not going to ask you to do lots of exercise with which you are uncomfortable. This plan is about healing your gut and making you feel better. With weight loss as an extra benefit.

There are many factors that contribute to a healthy body and mind and we cannot ignore exercise. Gentle exercise can help stimulate the gut and contribute to a healthy digestion. It will also help you de-stress, which will also help you feel better inside.

If you have a regular exercise routine (three times or more a week), you're doing great. Stick to what you're already doing. But if you find your work, commitments or health concerns stop you exercising regularly, then this is what I would suggest ...

Walk for half an hour at least three times a week. Yes, that's right – simply go for a walk. It would be even better if you tried to do this every day. Think about how or where you could do this. Is it getting off the bus at an earlier stop? A walk round the town at lunchtime? A stroll with the dog (or someone else's) at the end of the day?

Why is simple walking so beneficial?

Walking is a fantastic exercise for many reasons. Perhaps the most important is that it lowers your stress hormones. This not only makes you feel better but also encourages your body to burn fat, not sugar. Your metabolic response to walking means that each time you walk (or swim or do yoga) you are reducing your insulin resistance by a tiny bit and enhancing your ability to burn fat. You are also stretching out your intestinal system and giving gravity a helping hand, thus speeding up a sluggish digestion.

'Never dismiss walking as
"not proper exercise";
embrace and enjoy it.'

Part 2

THE 28-DAY PLAN

LET'S DO IT!

Here's a quick guide to the next 28 days. Don't worry, I'll guide you through every step of the way. For each day of the programme, you complete a **Gut-Health Diary** (see pages 101–28 for examples). It's really important that you allow yourself five minutes every morning, and again every evening, to fill in the diary. It is this that shows you the connections between food intolerances and gut symptoms. Be honest with yourself.

1	2	3	4	5	6	7
Rest and Restore	Rest and Restore	Rest and Restore	Rest and Restore	Rest and Restore	Rest and Restore	Rest and Restore
8	**9**	**10**	**11**	**12**	**13**	**14**
Introducing… Milk	Introducing… Milk	Introducing… Milk	Introducing… Red Meat	Introducing… Red Meat	Introducing… Red Meat	Rest or Adventure
15	**16**	**17**	**18**	**19**	**20**	**21**
Introducing… Nightshade	Introducing… Nightshade	Introducing… Nightshade	Rest or Adventure	Introducing… Gassy Veg	Introducing… Gassy Veg	Introducing… Gassy Veg
22	**23**	**24**	**25**	**26**	**27**	**28**
Rest or Adventure	Introducing… Wheat	Introducing… Wheat	Introducing… Wheat	Better Living	Better Living	Better Living

FOLLOWING THE PLAN

For each phase of the plan there is a huge variety of recipes you can use. **Step Up Recipes** are a great place to start. The Step Up Recipes are staple recipes that you can start in the Rest and Restore phase and then add extra ingredients for Introducing phases.

In the **Recipes** section, you'll find over eighty delicious recipes (over twenty for R&R alone). The recipes are divided into sections to match the phases of the plan. Each recipe also has an 'at a glance' guide to which food triggers (if any) it contains.

REST AND RESTORE

The plan starts with seven days of Rest and Restore (aka R&R). These seven days are vital to allow your gut to start to rebuild and recover.

How to do Rest and Restore
Start taking probiotics. Only eat safe foods. Banish all five triggers completely from your diet:

- Lactose (Milk)
- Red Meat
- Nightshade
- Gassy Veg
- Wheat

What happens within your gut during this phase?
We are trying to reduce the inflammation in your gut during this phase by cutting out all possible triggers. The surface of

your gut lining will start the slow process of rebuilding and becoming less porous.

Equally important is the addition of good bacteria in the form of probiotics. Adding probiotics improves the balance of gut bacteria by reducing the number of harmful bacteria.

What you should expect during this phase?

If you have other (non-gut) symptoms that you suspect are food- or gut-related, then you should see an improvement in these during the week. Because of the nature of gut bacteria, however, you might see discomfort and bloating actually increase during the Rest and Restore phase. Don't be disheartened. Think of this as the good bacteria starting to wage war against the build-up of years and years of bad bacteria. They might lose a couple of battles early on, but you've got more and more probiotics to put into action against the bad bacteria and eventually you will be victorious.

Expect to see bloating increase up to about days four to five, and start to slowly decrease after that. Track the measurements of your waistline (see page 100 for guidance) to plot changes to bloating within your gut. If this takes a bit longer, don't worry; this is perfectly normal. You just need a little patience.

Please don't start an Introducing phase until you are comfortable that the bloating has passed and your waistline measurement has not changed more than an inch in three days.

REST/ADVENTURE DAYS

We use the Rest/Adventure days to either (a) allow the body to recuperate after finding a moderate to severe trigger food or (b) to mix and match between already tested and cleared triggers. For example, the first Rest/Adventure day comes after the Milk and Red Meat Introducing phases. If you have given yourself the all-clear for both of these foodstuffs, you can eat them both in moderation on this day.

Rest Day

If you feel you have tested positive to a food intolerance during an Introducing phase, then this day will be a Rest Day.

On a Rest Day you simply go back to eating from the Rest and Restore plan. Even if you feel that some foods are OK from previous tests, do not eat them on this day. Keep it simple.

If one day is not enough to recover from a food to which you have found a strong intolerance, it is better to wait an extra day or two before continuing to the next phase.

Adventure Day

If you have given yourself the all-clear from one or more of the trigger food groups, you can food combine on this day and eat foods from any of your safe-food groups.

FOOD INTRODUCING PHASES

Each Introducing phase lasts for three days. On each day, a controlled amount of the foodstuff is added to your diet. This is isolated from any other possible triggers so that you do not cross-contaminate.

The order of the Introducing recipes is: Milk, Red Meat, Nightshade, Gas-inducing/Gassy Vegetables, Wheat and Gluten.

This leaves the most troublesome two, gassy vegetables and wheat, to the end so you have the best chance of tackling them head-on. They are also not likely to be linked. Two pairs of triggers exist. Milk and red meat are one pair; nightshade and gassy vegetables another. With a pair of triggers, if you have one it is *slightly* more likely that you have the other.

There are two important rules to follow during the Introducing phases. Firstly, do not eat any other trigger foods during this time. Even a little bit of a food that you think holds no issues can blur the lines and make a definitive result less likely.

And then, even more importantly, you must record, record, record. Make a note of every little change in your body – even if it's a red herring. When you reflect at the end of the three days you will have a definite score for your Intolerance:

Tolerant: Score 0 or 1. Can eat a moderate portion once a day with no symptoms.

Possibly Intolerant: Score 2 or 3. Some signs of symptoms when consuming a moderate portion.

Definitely Intolerant: Score 4 or 5. Show definite symptoms in the twenty-four hours following consumption of the food.

The first day is an isolated test, followed by twenty-four hours of symptom-checking. On the second day we increase the quantities and record symptoms again. This helps us differentiate between a minor or major intolerance. And finally, on day three we eat the same quantities as day two and we are testing for a build-up or an accumulation of the food. Is it safe to eat every day?

There is also the possibility that you won't finish the three days for an Introducing phase. The most likely reason for this is if you score Definitely Intolerant for Day One or Day Two, it would be counterproductive for you to continue this phase. You know you have an intolerance, and eating more of the food that caused it will just make your symptoms worse.

If this is the case, then you should return to Rest and Restore days for the rest of the phase. Your body will need forty-eight hours to recover from a food reaction.

DAY-BY-DAY GUIDE

Follow the day-by-day guide in conjunction witnh the **Gut-Health Diary** to record changes from Day 1 onwards.

DAYS 1–7: REST AND RESTORE YOUR GUT

The Rest and Restore (R&R) phase of the plan is the most restrictive in terms of what you can eat. Remember we are removing all five trigger foods: milk, red meat, nightshade, gassy veg, and wheat and gulten.

Take a look at the **Safe Foods** list (see pages 45–8) as well as the **Hero Foods** (pages 50–2) that you might need to buy in advance. Use the Step Up and R&R recipes to inspire you. These recipes should form the basis of what you eat during this phase.

1. Rest the gut
2. Only eat safe foods
3. Take probiotics
✓ Continue this phase for at least a week. The signal that you are ready to move on is three days with few or no symptoms.

- ✓ The length of time you spend in this phase will depend on the state of your gut lining and the balance of gut bacteria.
- ✓ If you want to spend longer on this phase or come back to it at any time then you should. This is your safe place.

DAYS 8–10: INTRODUCING … MILK

Milk lactose is introduced first into the programme. It is relatively easy to isolate from other trigger foods and therefore slightly easier for you to detect if you have a problem with milk lactose.

Lactose intolerance can be associated with sinus problems and skin conditions, particularly acne. If you suffer from either of these, then the likelihood of a lactose intolerance is slightly higher. Note also that there is some correlation between lactose intolerance and red meat intolerance, so having one could possibly suggest the other.

The Milk Test

Drink a glass of milk at around lunchtime or early afternoon. A glass of milk is 200–250ml, about 1 cup.

Check for changes in your symptoms and record them in your Gut-Health Diary twice daily:

- Just before bed
- The next morning

Day 8

Take the Milk Test at lunchtime. Record any changes in symptoms on the planner.

Day 9

The changes that could have occurred overnight from Day 1 to 2 give us the clearest indication of any intolerance. Take the time to consider any changes, even if they seem small. You should also record changes you felt during the night, even if they have now disappeared.

Milk Test Results

You can now see if you passed or failed the Milk Test. Look at your gut-health score for the evening of Day 8 and the morning of Day 9. The higher number is your Milk Test Score.

Milk Test Score: ....

If your Milk Test Score was:

    0 or 1: Lucky you. You probably are not intolerant to milk

    2 or 3: You may have an intolerance to milk. Further checks
        are necessary.

    4 or 5: You are definitely milk intolerant.

If your test results show you are definitely milk intolerant, then you should end the test here. Your Milk Intolerance Score will be 5 – Definitely Intolerant. You should now move on to a Rest Day. Allow your body to recover and if you have experienced some bloating, allow your tummy to return to normal before continuing with the next Introducing phase.

If your test results show that you are not intolerant to milk OR that you possibly have a milk intolerance, we continue with the second day of the Introducing phase.

Continuing Day 9 (Introducing Milk 2)

During Day 9, you should consume two portions of milk-based products. A portion could be:

- Milk on your cereal
- A glass of milk
- A pot of natural yogurt
- 3–4 cups of tea or coffee with milk
- A recipe from 'Introducing ... Milk' (see pages 176–80)

You just need to make sure you have two portions during the day. Record any changes in your symptoms.

Day 10

Unless your symptoms were very strong during Day 9 (in which case you should stop and mark yourself as 'Definitely Intolerant to Milk 5'), then Day 10 is very similar to Day 9. Eat or drink two or three portions of milk during the day and record your symptoms.

Milk Intolerance Score

You should work out your milk intolerance score the morning after the end of the Introducing Milk phase (i.e. Day 11). Look over your gut-health scores for all days included in the Introducing phase – that's Day 8, Day 9, Day 10 and the morning of Day 11.

If any of your scores were the result of another factor – eating another trigger food, excessive stress or tension, starting your period, etc. – discount this score.

Then take your highest score over the three days, morning or evening.

My Milk Intolerance Score ....

Intolerant: Score 4 or 5

Any food containing lactose can set off your intolerance and upset your stomach. You should avoid all milk, cream, yogurt and soft cheeses. Use of lactose-free milk is recommended. You will need to be careful about eating foods that you have not prepared yourself. Look out for milk powders and hidden milk in bread and biscuits, etc.

Mildly Intolerant: Score 2 or 3

You will have a reaction to milk sometimes. This is normally when you consume a lot of milk – a creamy dessert or an ice cream, for example. However, moderate quantities of milk can be consumed daily. Stick to one portion a day and you should be fine. Be aware that if you are feeling under the weather or stressed, or your gut health has deteriorated for other reasons, then your milk intolerance may temporarily increase.

In all cases, if you feel that you are more sensitive to milk for any reason, remove it from your diet for at least forty-eight hours (or up to a week depending on your circumstances) until all symptoms have passed. This will reset your system and you will be back to being 'Mildly Intolerant' again.

Tolerant: Score 0 or 1

You do not have a problem with milk or lactose. You should drink and eat it freely.

DAYS 11–13: INTRODUCING ... RED MEAT

We go straight on to this phase after finishing the milk phase. There are not enough food groups to allow us to be adventurous. The exception would be if you discovered a milk intolerance and therefore needed to leave yourself a day or two to reset before attempting this phase.

The Red Meat Test

Eat a small (less than 125g/4oz) beef or pork steak. The meat should be lean and thoroughly cooked. It is best to eat the red meat at lunchtime with potatoes or rice and some safe vegetables or salad. If it's simpler for you, then you can eat the red meat as part of an early dinner, but be aware that if you do have a reaction to the red meat, the later you eat it, the more likely it is to disturb your sleep.

Day 11

Take the Red Meat Test at lunchtime or dinner time and record any changes to your gut health in the evening just before bed and first thing the next morning.

Day 12

You can get your Red Meat Test Results as soon as you have filled in your daily planner for the morning of Day 12. Be aware that if you have a reaction to red meat it could be more extreme than you might experience with other food triggers. This is because the reaction is more likely to be bacterial rather than related to the gut lining. Don't despair, probiotics will reduce this reaction, and a red-meat intolerance is the most likely to be fixed or improved by continued use of probiotics.

Red Meat Test Results

You can now see if you passed or failed the Red Meat Test. Look at your gut-health score for the evening of Day 11 and the morning of Day 12. The higher number is your Red Meat Test Score.

> Red Meat Test Score: ....
>
> If your Red Meat Test score was:
>   0 or 1: Lucky you. You probably are not intolerant to red meat.
>   2 or 3: You may have an intolerance to red meat. Further checks are necessary.
>   4 or 5: You are definitely red-meat intolerant.

If your test results show you are definitely red meat intolerant, then you should end the test here. Your Red Meat Intolerance Score will be 5 – Definitely Intolerant. You should now move on to a Rest Day. Allow your body to recover and if you have experienced some bloating, allow your tummy to return to normal before continuing the next Introducing phase.

If your test results show that you are not intolerant to red meat OR that you possibly have a red meat intolerance, we continue with the second day of the Introducing phase.

Continuing Day 12 (Introducing Red Meat Day 2)

Repeat the Red Meat Test or use a recipe from Introducing ... Red Meat (see pages 181–7). If you are eating beef steak, and prefer it a little bit pink, this is a good test for today. Make sure you consume at least as much red meat as Day 11, preferably a little bit more. Lamb and other red meats are also allowed. You can add ham and bacon, etc., too, but make sure at least one generous portion of red meat is unprocessed.

Day 13

Unless your symptoms were very strong during Day 12 (in which case you should stop and mark yourself as 'Definitely Intolerant to Red Meat 5'), then Day 13 is very similar to Day 12. Eat one or two portions of red meat (at least one portion being unprocessed) during the day and record your symptoms.

Red Meat Intolerance Score

You should work out your Red Meat Intolerance Score the morning after the end of the Red Meat Introducing phase (i.e. Day 14). Look over your gut-health scores for all days of this Introducing phase – that's Day 11, Day 12, Day 13 and the morning of Day 14.

If any of your scores had another factor – eating another trigger food, excessive stress or tension, starting your period, etc. – discount this score. Then take your highest score over the three days, morning or evening.

My Red Meat Intolerance Score ....

Intolerant: Score 4 or 5

Any food containing red meat can set off your intolerance and upset your stomach. You should avoid all red meat, including minced beef, ham, bacon and sausages.

Mildly Intolerant: Score 2 or 3

You will have a reaction to red meat sometimes. This is normally when you consume a lot of unprocessed red meat – a big, juicy steak, for example. However, moderate quantities of red meat, both pro- cessed and unprocessed, can be consumed daily. Stick to one portion a day and you should be fine. Be aware that if you are feeling under the weather or stressed, or your gut health has deteriorated for other reasons, then your red meat intolerance may temporarily increase.

In all cases if you feel that you are more sensitive to red meat for any reason, remove it from your diet for at least forty-eight hours (or up to a week depending on your circumstances) until all symptoms have passed. This will reset your system and you will be back to being 'Mildly Intolerant' again.

Not Intolerant: Score 0 or 1

You do not have a problem with red meat. You should eat it freely.

DAY 14: REST DAY OR ADVENTURE DAY

Depending on how your stomach and gut feels, you should either have a Rest Day (and eat carefully and sensibly from the Safe Foods list (see pages 45–8) and Recipes section) or have an Adventure Day where you can eat both milk and red meat if you feel you are not intolerant to either. Keep recording the food you eat and any changes in your gut health during this time.

DAYS 15–17 INTRODUCING ...
NIGHTSHADE

Only when you are comfortable that you don't have any residual symptoms or bloating from the Milk and Red Meat Introducing phases should you start introducing nightshade into your diet.

There are two tests for nightshade: The Tomato Test and The Chilli Test. These should be taken on Day 15 and Day 16 respectively.

Nightshade intolerance is most likely to be a result of an accumulation of too much nightshade. Think of it as a very mild poison. A small quantity should be fine, but if you eat it in huge amounts, or when your stomach is already delicate, it will cause a reaction. For this reason we test nightshade slightly differently to milk and red meat.

The Tomato Test

Eat one medium to large tomato at lunchtime or as part of an early dinner. This can be as simple as taking a fresh tomato and eating it like an apple. Here's a tip! A tomato at room temperature has more flavour than if it comes straight from the fridge. You can also eat your tomato as part of a simple salad.

The Chilli Test

Chillies can irritate the stomach lining in a slightly different way to tomatoes, so we test this the day after The Tomato Test. As chillies are often eaten in combination with tomatoes, you can eat chilli and tomato together as part of this test. Eat either a fresh chilli (washed and carefully deseeded) as part of a cooked meal or add a teaspoon of mild chilli powder or paprika to a dish. The dish can contain tomatoes.

If you don't like hot and spicy food, sprinkle paprika on a tomato salad as this adds the least heat.

Day 15

Take The Tomato Test on previous page. Record any changes as they happen. Unless you have a very strong reaction (gut-health symptoms 5) you should continue to Day 16.

Day 16

Take The Chilli Test on previous page. And eat one to two portions of tomatoes, aubergine (eggplant) or (bell) peppers.

Day 17

Repeat Day 16, increasing quantities of all types of nightshade if you feel able. Write down all nightshade foods eaten and the quantity consumed.

You can get your Nightshade Intolerance Score as soon as you have filled in your daily planner for the morning of Day 18. Remember that nightshade is likely to be cumulative. So the number of portions and the build-up of quantities over time should be carefully recorded.

Nightshade Intolerance Score

Look at your gut-health score over the three days of Introducing Nightshade. Don't forget the morning of Day 18. The highest number is your Nightshade Test Score.

Nightshade Intolerance Score: ....

Intolerant: Score 4 or 5

Any food containing tomato, peppers or any form of chilli (including red spices) can set off your intolerance and upset your stomach. You should avoid all spicy food and steer clear of tomatoes and peppers. You may find that you can occasionally eat a little bit of nightshade in the future. But introduce it very slowly after a long period of safe eating.

Mildly Intolerant: Score 2 or 3

You will have a reaction to larger amounts of nightshade. Stick to one portion a day and you should be fine. You will be more intolerant to foods containing tomatoes and chillies together, so be extra careful with spicy tomato dishes. Be aware that if you are feeling under the weather or stressed, or your gut health has deteriorated for other reasons, then your nightshade intolerance may temporarily increase.

Not Intolerant: Score 0 or 1

You do not have a problem with nightshade.

DAY 18: REST DAY OR ADVENTURE DAY

Depending on how your stomach and gut feel, you should either have a Rest Day (eat carefully and sensibly from the Safe Foods list (see page 45–8) and Recipes section) or have an

Adventure Day where you can eat milk, red meat and nightshade. There are Adventure Day recipes for mixing up these three food triggers. Keep recording the food you eat and any changes during this time so that you can spot changes in your gut-health quickly.

DAYS 19–21: INTRODUCING … GASSY VEGETABLES

Now we get on to the even trickier foods. Onions and garlic get into so many of the dishes we eat. They are especially problematic because even the smallest quantity can trigger a reaction. It is also the most common food trigger and many people with sensitive digestive systems have some kind of reaction to gassy foods.

Foods containing Gassy Veg

Onions	Cabbage
Garlic	Beans
Broccoli	Lentils
Cauliflower	Chickpeas
Kale	

The Hummus Test

Hummus is a great way to test a gassy veg intolerance in a controlled fashion because it contains both chickpeas and garlic. You can make a batch on the first day and then use it to continue testing on the other days of this Introducing phase.

Two-minute Hummus

Makes 4 portions
1 x 400g (14oz) tin chickpeas, rinsed and drained
1 garlic clove, peeled
1 tbsp extra-virgin olive oil
1 heaped tsp peanut butter
juice of 1 lemon
salt and freshly ground pepper
a little extra water, if needed

The easiest way to make this is to use a food processor or blender – just chuck in all the ingredients and blitz.

If you don't have a blender, crush the chickpeas with the back of a fork and use a garlic press to crush the garlic. Place in a bowl with the olive oil, slightly watered down peanut butter, lemon juice and salt and pepper and continue to stir and crush with the back of a fork until you get a rough paste.

Day 19

Make a batch of the hummus on the first day. Divide it into quarters and eat the first portion at lunchtime today. It's important that you eat it at lunchtime, as with gassy veg intolerance you are most likely to get stomach cramps overnight and we want to avoid that if at all possible.

Record your symptoms carefully as soon as they appear. Remember it is the gas released from the gassy veg when it is digested that causes the problem, so symptoms can start to appear within a couple of hours and continue for up to twenty-four. The most likely symptoms are cramps and wind.

Day 20

The changes that could have occurred overnight from Days 19 to 20 give us the clearest indication of any intolerance. Take the time to consider any changes even if they seem small. You should also record changes you felt in the night, even if they have now disappeared.

Gassy Veg (Hummus) Test Results

You can now see if you passed or failed the Gassy Veg Test. Look at your gut-health score for the evening of Day 19 and the morning of Day 20. The higher number is your Gassy Veg Test Score.

> Gassy Veg Test Score: ....
>
> If your gassy veg test score was:
>   0 or 1: Lucky you. You probably are not intolerant to gassy veg.
>   2 or 3: You may have an intolerance to gassy veg. Further
>   checks are necessary.
>   4 or 5: You are definitely intolerant to gassy veg.

If your test results show you are definitely gassy veg intolerant, then you should end the test here. Your Gassy Veg Intolerance Score will be 5 – Definitely Intolerant. You should now move on to a Rest Day. Allow your body to recover and if you have experienced some bloating, allow your tummy to return to normal before continuing the next Introducing phase.

If your test results show that you are not intolerant to gassy veg OR that you possibly have a gassy veg intolerance, we continue with the second day of the Introducing phase.

Continuing Day 20 (Introducing Gassy Veg Day 2)

During Day 20, you should consume gassy veg at lunch and dinner. One portion could be a slightly larger serving of

Two-minute Hummus and the second portion should be onion or some description. Take a look at introducing ... Gassy Veg recipes (see pages 208–14) for some ideas. Record any changes in your symptoms.

Day 21

Unless your symptoms were very strong during Day 20 (in which case you should stop and mark yourself as 'Definitely Intolerant to Gassy Veg 5') then Day 21 is very similar to Day 20. Eat two portions of gassy veg over lunch and dinner and record your symptoms.

Gassy Veg Intolerance Score

You should work out your Gassy Veg Intolerance Score the morning after the end of the Introducing Gassy Veg phase (i.e. Day 22). Look over your gut-health scores for all days of this Introducing phase – that's Day 19, Day 20, Day 21 and the morning of Day 22.

Take your highest score over the three days, morning or evening. This is your Gassy Veg Intolerance Score.

My Gassy Veg Intolerance Score: ....

Intolerant: Score 4 or 5

Avoid any foods containing any form of onions, garlic, gassy veg, beans, lentils or chickpeas. Even a tiny amount of these foods can set off your intolerance and upset your stomach. You will need to be careful eating foods that you have not prepared yourself. Look out for trigger words like 'onion' and 'garlic', in any form – powder, extract, flavour, etc. Be aware that all stock powders and fresh shop-bought stock will contain onion in some form or other.

Mildly Intolerant: Score 2 or 3

You will have a reaction to larger quantities of gassy veg. A small amount, like a stock powder or one clove of garlic in a meal for four, should not trigger your intolerance. Keep clear of raw onion or dishes with onion or garlic in the title. Avoid all lentils, beans and chickpeas.

In all cases, if you are feeling more delicate remove gassy veg from your diet FIRST (before any other possible triggers).

Tolerant: Score 0 or 1

You do not have a problem with gassy veg. Note that most people, even without this sensitivity, will get a gut reaction to a hot, spicy curry due to the massive combination of lots of onions, garlic and chilli.

DAY 22: REST DAY OR ADVENTURE DAY

Unless you're feeling really confident, make this a Rest Day in preparation for the gluten and wheat to come.

DAYS 23–25: INTRODUCING ... WHEAT

Like gassy veg, wheat is a tricky beast. It's hard to pinpoint as wheat gets into so many of our favourite foods. Unlike gassy veg, the symptoms of wheat intolerance are most likely to be related to bloating or to other (non-gut) symptoms, such as skin complaints like eczema and acne.

For that reason, *before* we introduce wheat we need to consider whether we've seen improvements in other conditions during the programme so far. We are now three weeks into the plan, so you will have been wheat-free for all of that time. This allows you a unique opportunity to see what effect being wheat-free has on the rest of your body.

Check for Improvements in Non-gut Symptoms before Wheat Introduction

At this stage, it's worth referring back to your Initial Gut Assessment and reviewing your Inflammation scores (Questions 4–8, page 26), then and comparing them with now.

4. Do you have skin complaints? For example, itchy skin, rashes, eczema, rosacea, acne, hives, psoriasis.

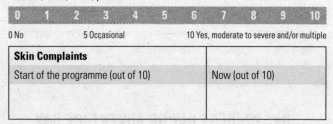

| 0 | 1 | 2 | 3 | 4 | 5 | 6 | 7 | 8 | 9 | 10 |

0 No   5 Occasional   10 Yes, moderate to severe and/or multiple

Skin Complaints	
Start of the programme (out of 10)	Now (out of 10)

5. Do you have hay fever, dust or pet allergies?

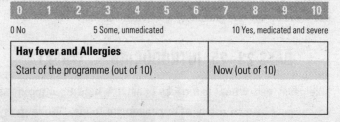

| 0 | 1 | 2 | 3 | 4 | 5 | 6 | 7 | 8 | 9 | 10 |

0 No   5 Some, unmedicated   10 Yes, medicated and severe

Hay fever and Allergies	
Start of the programme (out of 10)	Now (out of 10)

6. Do you experience joint pain or unexplained muscle pain?

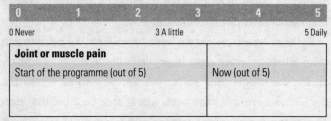

| 0 | 1 | 2 | 3 | 4 | 5 |

0 Never   3 A little   5 Daily

Joint or muscle pain	
Start of the programme (out of 5)	Now (out of 5)

7. Do you suffer from frequent sinus pain or other sinus-related issues?

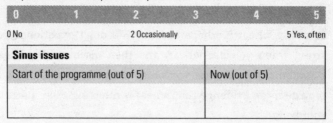

0	1	2	3	4	5
0 No		2 Occasionally			5 Yes, often

Sinus issues	
Start of the programme (out of 5)	Now (out of 5)

8. Do you get problems such as brain fog, chronic headaches, anxiety?

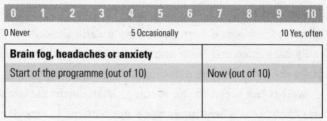

0	1	2	3	4	5	6	7	8	9	10
0 Never					5 Occasionally					10 Yes, often

Brain fog, headaches or anxiety	
Start of the programme (out of 10)	Now (out of 10)

By comparing the results in numbers you will be able to see what, if any, effect wheat has had on other parts of your body. A significant improvement in these symptoms is indicated by a change of at least two points in two or more of these questions.

> Do you have a significant improvement in Inflammation Symptoms?
>
> ☐ YES   ☐ NO

If you can't see any significant improvement between the start of the programme and now, then you are less likely to have a wheat intolerance. If you see quite big changes in at least two of these markers, then this significantly increases your risk of having an intolerance to wheat. There's no on–off switch for these, which makes it really hard to see what difference wheat is making to your overall health. If you go back to eating wheat (perhaps because you don't experience gut stress when you eat wheat) and then discover that these symptoms worsen after you finish the programme, this will provide more evidence that wheat is affecting other parts of your body.

The Bread Test

The test for wheat is beautifully simple. Eat a slice of bread/a roll/a cake (nice and fresh and delicious – you might as well make the most of it!) as part of your evening meal.

We eat the bread in the evening, as stomach cramps are less likely with wheat intolerance. But bloating is very likely. The best time to measure this is first thing in the morning after having had wheat the night before.

Day 23

At the start of the day take a waistline (bloating) measurement and record it in your Gut-Health Diary. This will be important for comparison at the start of Day 24.

Take The Bread Test. Record any changes as they happen. Unless you have a very strong reaction (gut-health symptoms 5) you should continue to Day 24.

Day 24

Check your waistline again this morning. Has it increased since yesterday morning? This measurement is the best way to see if the wheat has resulted in bloating.

Repeat The Bread Test. You can have two portions of wheat, either both in the evening or one at lunch and one as part of the evening meal. One wheat portion could be pasta.

Day 25

Again, check your waistline measurement and watch for any changes.

Repeat Day 24, increasing quantities if you feel able.

You can get your Wheat Intolerance Score as soon as you have filled in your daily planner for the morning of Day 26. Remember that wheat intolerance is likely to be cumulative. So the number of portions and the build-up of quantities over time should be carefully recorded.

Wheat Intolerance Score

Look at your gut-health score over the three days of introducing wheat. Don't forget the morning of Day 26. The highest number is your Wheat Intolerance Score.

Wheat Intolerance Score: ....

Look again at the Inflammation questions. If you answered YES to the question 'Do you have a significant improvement in Inflammation Symptoms?' then **ADD ONE** to your wheat intolerance score to arrive at your adjusted score.

Adjusted (Final) Wheat Intolerance Score: ....

Intolerant: Score 4 or 5

Any food containing wheat is an issue for you. That includes bread, pasta, cakes and even small quantities of wheat. You'll need to check the packaging on shop-bought items for wheat and gluten. As wheat and gluten are considered allergens they are often highlighted in bold to help you.

You may not be intolerant to gluten that comes in other forms to wheat. You can test this separately by trying foods containing barley gluten. The good news is that this includes beer! Malt extract is also a great food to try for gluten intolerance, or barley flakes.

Mildly Intolerant: Score 2 or 3

You will have a reaction to larger amounts of wheat. The key to control is to keep the portion size down. Strictly one meal a day containing wheat and you might be OK, although if you are mildly intolerant you may find your inflammation symptoms slowly increasing.

If you find that your inflammation comes back with a small amount of wheat, then remove wheat entirely until the symptoms disappear.

Then carefully (using the three-day plan) introduce barley gluten in the form of beer or malt extract. There is a fantastic muesli recipe in the Introducing ... Wheat and Gluten recipes (see page 216) that includes barley flakes that would be a great gluten test.

You might also want to test Kamut flour (again, there are some great recipes for Kamut bread and rolls in the Recipes section) as this is less likely to cause bloating and inflammation symptoms than normal bread.

Tolerant: Score 0 or 1

You do not have a problem with wheat.

DAYS 26–28: BETTER LIVING FOR YOU

The last few days of the programme are for you to take stock of what you have learned so far and to do a little bit of extra testing based on your own sensitivities. This will help you fill in any final gaps in your knowledge surrounding your own specific set of circumstances. For example, perhaps you tested nightshade during your period and think this might have skewed your results slightly. Or you went to a party on the first weekend of the plan, may have eaten some wheat and think this may have had an impact on your milk score.

All these things (and more) are worth considering in order to get the best picture of how your gut behaves.

In the Recipes section, you'll find the final chapter consists of recipes for food combining. At last, you can have gassy veg and nightshade together again! The idea is for you to combine two or three trigger foods at once rather than all five. This allows you to continue to track your symptoms for the last three days just in case you get a few rogue elements.

The impact of food on your gut is not an exact science and a food can have no effect one day and a significant effect on another.

The **Gut-Health Diary** in the following chapter allows you to pick up patterns from the foods you eat and reach your own conclusions about what is best for you.

The final tool in your gut-health assessment is the **28-Day Review** (see page 129). You should complete this during the **Better Living for You** phase. It will bring together what you have learned over the 28-Day Plan. Keep this review for when you forget about the detail of the plan. You could even take a photo of it with your phone for reference later.

'The 28-Day Review is a unique jigsaw for your gut health and you can use it to continue your own gut-improvement journey.'

LOOKING FORWARD, NEVER BACK

If you've completed the plan, then firstly CONGRATULATIONS. Give yourself a huge pat on the back. You deserve it. You have gained a far greater understanding of your body and your digestive system. Do you feel better? Do you glow? Have you lost weight?

You have taken a massive step forward in mastering your own digestive health. But Rome wasn't built in a day. And decades of digestive destruction cannot be fixed in a month. So there is still a long way to go to attain gut perfection.

You now have the tools – your 28-Day Review, probiotics, gut-friendly recipes – to keep improving your gut-health into the future.

GUT-HEALTH DIARY

Use this diary to record how you feel, how your tummy feels and what you have eaten during each day of the 28-Day Gut-Health Plan.

Give yourself five minutes each morning and again at night to make a note of the foods that you eat and monitor your symptoms.

Remember, a printable version of **The Gut-Health Diary** can be downloaded (for free!) from **www.52recipes.co.uk/28G**.

The first entry is just a sample that I have completed myself. Your **Gut-Health Diary** is just for you. **Please be honest with yourself**. You don't have to justify it. No one is judging you. But honesty will help you better understand your gut.

SAMPLE DAY
Thursday (19) Gassy Veg 1 (eek)

Morning

Last night I slept... *Quite badly. I don't know what it was though. My tummy feels OK.*

This morning I feel... *OK. A bit tired.*

My tummy feels... *A bit bloated but nothing major. Gurgly?*

I would score my gut health as   0   1   **2**   3   4   5
(0 – no symptoms, 5 – severe symptoms)

Yesterday I... *Had a glass of wine. Did it affect my sleep?*
(which may be affecting my symptoms today)

My waistline (bloating) is   UP   DOWN   **THE SAME**

Notes (including optional weigh-in) *Gonna blame the wine. It was more than a glass!*

Evening

Today I ate:

Morning   *Chia Choc Granola + lactose-free milk. Lots of tea.*

Lunch   *Hummus and gluten-free bread and cucumber. Chocolate. More tea.*

Evening   *Egg-fried rice and prawns. Chocolate. White wine.*

My tummy feels... *Fine*

I would score my gut health as   **0**   1   2   3   4   5
(0 – no symptoms, 5 – severe symptoms)

Opportunities for Improvement   *Wine affects my sleep and makes me hungry! (Stop drinking wine!)*

Wins   *Maybe I'm not gassy veg intolerant??*

HOW TO RATE YOUR SYMPTOMS?

Sometimes it's hard to compare like with like when it comes to your symptoms. It's easy to forget or confuse one day with another. And it's virtually impossible to tally the foods you eat with your symptoms. That's why it's important to score your symptoms for the day, as well as making a note of the foods that you eat.

You should always track your symptoms first thing in the morning and last thing at night.

Look at the following symptoms and decide which, if any, was worst:

- Stomach cramps
- Constipation
- Diarrhoea
- Bloating (use the waistline measurement)
- Wind

Then give the **worst symptom** a score between 0 and 5. A score of 5 is the most severe and a score of 0 means no symptoms at all. Any score of 3 or above suggests you need to look at the foods eaten in the last 24 hours.

Use the following guide to best judge your symptoms:

5 – Severe. Disrupted sleep. Major impact on your day. Visible bloating. Your gut is a constant source of worry.

4 – Moderately severe. Some disruption to your sleep and your day. You feel bad but can remember other recent days that were worse.

3 – Moderate. Tossing and turning in your sleep but it doesn't keep you awake. Annoying but manageable.

2 – Mild to Moderate. No sleep disruption but you feel it when you wake up. You worry that the symptoms might get worse but actually they don't.

1 – Mild. There's still something going on in your gut. But it's not causing you any problems.

0 – No symptoms. Regular bowel movements. No pain. No bloating.

HOW TO UNDERSTAND BLOATING

Measuring your waistline gives an objective measure of the size of the stomach and helps you see if your gut is bloated or inflamed. It can be used on its own or in conjunction with your body weight. Don't feel you need to track your waistline every day, but you should be consistent with the time of day. The best time to do this is first thing in the morning. Bloating tends to appear overnight and can last all day.

If you want to remember your weight changes over the programme, there is also room to record that information in the diary but it is optional.

To measure your waistline

Place three fingers directly below your belly button. You should measure around your waist from the bottom of your third finger, or 5cm/2in below your belly button. This means you are always measuring exactly the same part of your body. Place the measuring tape around your waist to meet at the same point at the front. Do not breathe in or overly tighten the tape. Remember you are measuring changes in your body, not in comparison to anybody else.

DAY 1: R&R..

Morning

Last night I slept... ....
....

This morning I feel... ....

My tummy feels... ....

I would score my gut health as   0   1   2   3   4   5
(0 – no symptoms, 5 – severe symptoms)

Yesterday I... ....
(which may be affecting my symptoms today)

My waistline (bloating) is   UP   DOWN   THE SAME

Notes (including optional weigh-in) ....

Evening

Today's food:

   Morning   ....
....

   Lunch   ....
....

   Evening   ....

My tummy feels... ....

I would score my gut health as   0   1   2   3   4   5
(0 – no symptoms, 5 – severe symptoms)

Opportunities for improvement: ....
....

Wins   ....

DAY 2: R&R ....

Morning

Last night I slept... ....
....

This morning I feel... ....

My tummy feels... ....

I would score my gut health as   0   1   2   3   4   5
(0 – no symptoms, 5 – severe symptoms)

Yesterday I... ....
(which may be affecting my symptoms today)

My waistline (bloating) is   UP   DOWN   THE SAME

Notes (including optional weigh-in) ....

Evening

Today's food:

    Morning   ....
....

    Lunch   ....
....

    Evening   ....

My tummy feels... ....

I would score my gut health as   0   1   2   3   4   5
(0 – no symptoms, 5 – severe symptoms)

Opportunities for improvement...
....

Wins   ....

DAY 3: R&R ....

Morning

Last night I slept... ....
....

This morning I feel... ....

My tummy feels... ....

I would score my gut health as   0   1   2   3   4   5
(0 – no symptoms, 5 – severe symptoms)

Yesterday I... ....
(which may be affecting my symptoms today)

My waistline (bloating) is   UP   DOWN   THE SAME

Notes (including optional weigh-in) ....

Evening

Today's food:

    Morning   ....
....

    Lunch   ....
....

    Evening   ....

My tummy feels... ....

I would score my gut health as   0   1   2   3   4   5
(0 – no symptoms, 5 – severe symptoms)

Opportunities for improvement...
....

Wins   ....

DAY 4: R&R

Morning

Last night I slept… ....

....

This morning I feel… ....

My tummy feels… ....

I would score my gut health as   0   1   2   3   4   5
(0 – no symptoms, 5 – severe symptoms)

Yesterday I… ....
(which may be affecting my symptoms today)

My waistline (bloating) is   UP   DOWN   THE SAME

Notes (including optional weigh-in) ....

Evening

Today's food:

    Morning   ....

....

    Lunch   ....

....

    Evening   ....

My tummy feels… ....

I would score my gut health as   0   1   2   3   4   5
(0 – no symptoms, 5 – severe symptoms)

Opportunities for improvement..

....

Wins ....

DAY 5: R&R

Morning

Last night I slept... ....

....

This morning I feel... ....

My tummy feels... ....

I would score my gut health as   0   1   2   3   4   5
(0 – no symptoms, 5 – severe symptoms)

Yesterday I... ....
(which may be affecting my symptoms today)

My waistline (bloating) is   UP   DOWN   THE SAME

Notes (including optional weigh-in) ....

Evening

Today's food:

Morning   ....

....

Lunch   ....

....

Evening   ....

My tummy feels... ....

I would score my gut health as   0   1   2   3   4   5
(0 – no symptoms, 5 – severe symptoms)

Opportunities for improvement...

....

Wins   ....

DAY 6: R&R

Morning

Last night I slept... ....
....

This morning I feel... ....

My tummy feels... ....

I would score my gut health as   0   1   2   3   4   5
(0 – no symptoms, 5 – severe symptoms)

Yesterday I... ....
(which may be affecting my symptoms today)

My waistline (bloating) is   UP   DOWN   THE SAME

Notes (including optional weigh-in) ....

Evening

Today's food:
     Morning   ....
                          ....
     Lunch   ....
                          ....
     Evening   ....

My tummy feels... ....

I would score my gut health as   0   1   2   3   4   5
(0 – no symptoms, 5 – severe symptoms)

Opportunities for improvement..
....

Wins   ....

DAY 7: R&R ....

Morning

Last night I slept... ....
....

This morning I feel... ....

My tummy feels... ....

I would score my gut health as   0   1   2   3   4   5
(0 – no symptoms, 5 – severe symptoms)

Yesterday I... ....
(which may be affecting my symptoms today)

My waistline (bloating) is   UP   DOWN   THE SAME

Notes (including optional weigh-in) ....

Evening

Today's food:

    Morning   ....
....

    Lunch   ....
....

    Evening   ....

My tummy feels... ....

I would score my gut health as   0   1   2   3   4   5
(0 – no symptoms, 5 – severe symptoms)

Opportunities for improvement...
....

Wins   ....

DAY 8: INTRODUCING MILK 1 ....

Morning

Last night I slept... ....
....

This morning I feel... ....

My tummy feels... ....

I would score my gut health as   0   1   2   3   4   5
(0 – no symptoms, 5 – severe symptoms)

Yesterday I... ....
(which may be affecting my symptoms today)

My waistline (bloating) is   UP   DOWN   THE SAME

Notes (including optional weigh-in) ....

Evening

Today's food:

    Morning   ....
                         ....

    Lunch   ....
                         ....

    Evening   ....

My tummy feels... ....

I would score my gut health as   0   1   2   3   4   5
(0 – no symptoms, 5 – severe symptoms)

Opportunities for improvement...
....

Wins   ....

DAY 9: INTRODUCING MILK 2

Morning
Last night I slept… ....
....

This morning I feel… ....

My tummy feels… ....

I would score my gut health as   0   1   2   3   4   5
(0 – no symptoms, 5 – severe symptoms)

Yesterday I… ....
(which may be affecting my symptoms today)

My waistline (bloating) is   UP   DOWN   THE SAME

Notes (including optional weigh-in) ....

Evening
Today's food:

    Morning ....
....

    Lunch ....
....

    Evening ....

My tummy feels… ....

I would score my gut health as   0   1   2   3   4   5
(0 – no symptoms, 5 – severe symptoms)

Opportunities for improvement...
....

Wins ....

DAY 10: INTRODUCING MILK 3

Morning

Last night I slept… ....

....

This morning I feel… ....

My tummy feels… ....

I would score my gut health as   0   1   2   3   4   5
(0 – no symptoms, 5 – severe symptoms)

Yesterday I… ....
(which may be affecting my symptoms today)

My waistline (bloating) is   UP   DOWN   THE SAME

Notes (including optional weigh-in) ....

Evening

Today's food:

    Morning   ....

    ....

    Lunch   ....

    ....

    Evening   ....

My tummy feels… ....

I would score my gut health as   0   1   2   3   4   5
(0 – no symptoms, 5 – severe symptoms)

Opportunities for improvement ....

....

Wins   ....

DAY 11: INTRODUCING RED MEAT 1

Morning

Last night I slept… ....

....

This morning I feel… ....

My tummy feels… ....

I would score my gut health as   0   1   2   3   4   5
(0 – no symptoms, 5 – severe symptoms)

Yesterday I… ....
(which may be affecting my symptoms today)

My waistline (bloating) is   UP   DOWN   THE SAME

Notes (including optional weigh-in) ....

Evening

Today's food:

    Morning   ....

....

    Lunch   ....

....

    Evening   ....

My tummy feels… ....

I would score my gut health as   0   1   2   3   4   5
(0 – no symptoms, 5 – severe symptoms)

Opportunities for improvement ....

....

Wins   ....

DAY 12: INTRODUCING RED MEAT 2

Morning

Last night I slept… ....
....

This morning I feel… ....

My tummy feels… ....

I would score my gut health as   0   1   2   3   4   5
(0 – no symptoms, 5 – severe symptoms)

Yesterday I… ....
(which may be affecting my symptoms today)

My waistline (bloating) is   UP   DOWN   THE SAME

Notes (including optional weigh-in) ....

Evening

Today's food:

    Morning   ....
....

    Lunch   ....
....

    Evening   ....

My tummy feels… ....

I would score my gut health as   0   1   2   3   4   5
(0 – no symptoms, 5 – severe symptoms)

Opportunities for improvement..
....

Wins   ....

DAY 13: INTRODUCING RED MEAT 3 ....

Morning

Last night I slept... ....
....

This morning I feel... ....

My tummy feels... ....

I would score my gut health as   0   1   2   3   4   5
(0 – no symptoms, 5 – severe symptoms)

Yesterday I... ....
(which may be affecting my symptoms today)

My waistline (bloating) is   UP   DOWN   THE SAME

Notes (including optional weigh-in) ....

Evening

Today's food:

    Morning   ....
....

    Lunch   ....
....

    Evening   ....

My tummy feels... ....

I would score my gut health as   0   1   2   3   4   5
(0 – no symptoms, 5 – severe symptoms)

Opportunities for improvement...
....

Wins   ....

DAY 14: REST DAY OR ADVENTURE DAY

Morning

Last night I slept… ....
....

This morning I feel… ....

My tummy feels… ....

I would score my gut health as   0   1   2   3   4   5
(0 – no symptoms, 5 – severe symptoms)

Yesterday I… ....
(which may be affecting my symptoms today)

My waistline (bloating) is   UP   DOWN   THE SAME

Notes (including optional weigh-in) ....

Evening

Today's food:

Morning   ....
....

Lunch   ....
....

Evening   ....

My tummy feels… ....

I would score my gut health as   0   1   2   3   4   5
(0 – no symptoms, 5 – severe symptoms)

Opportunities for improvement...
....

Wins   ....

DAY 15: INTRODUCING NIGHTSHADE 1 ....

Morning

Last night I slept... ....
....

This morning I feel... ....

My tummy feels... ....

I would score my gut health as   0   1   2   3   4   5
(0 – no symptoms, 5 – severe symptoms)

Yesterday I... ....
(which may be affecting my symptoms today)

My waistline (bloating) is   UP   DOWN   THE SAME

Notes (including optional weigh-in) ....

Evening

Today's food:

    Morning   ....
....

    Lunch   ....
....

    Evening   ....

My tummy feels... ....

I would score my gut health as   0   1   2   3   4   5
(0 – no symptoms, 5 – severe symptoms)

Opportunities for improvement...
....

Wins   ....

DAY 16: INTRODUCING NIGHTSHADE 2

Morning

Last night I slept… ....

....

This morning I feel… ....

My tummy feels… ....

I would score my gut health as   0   1   2   3   4   5
(0 – no symptoms, 5 – severe symptoms)

Yesterday I… ....
(which may be affecting my symptoms today)

My waistline (bloating) is   UP   DOWN   THE SAME

Notes (including optional weigh-in) ....

Evening

Today's food:

    Morning   ....

....

    Lunch   ....

....

    Evening   ....

My tummy feels… ....

I would score my gut health as   0   1   2   3   4   5
(0 – no symptoms, 5 – severe symptoms)

Opportunities for improvement ....

....

Wins ....

DAY 17: INTRODUCING NIGHTSHADE 3

Morning

Last night I slept… ....

....

This morning I feel… ....

My tummy feels… ....

I would score my gut health as   0   1   2   3   4   5
(0 – no symptoms, 5 – severe symptoms)

Yesterday I… ....
(which may be affecting my symptoms today)

My waistline (bloating) is   UP   DOWN   THE SAME

Notes (including optional weigh-in) ....

Evening

Today's food:

  Morning ....

....

  Lunch ....

....

  Evening ....

My tummy feels… ....

I would score my gut health as   0   1   2   3   4   5
(0 – no symptoms, 5 – severe symptoms)

Opportunities for improvement...

....

Wins ....

DAY 18: REST DAY OR ADVENTURE DAY ....

Morning

Last night I slept... ....
....

This morning I feel... ....

My tummy feels... ....

I would score my gut health as   0   1   2   3   4   5
(0 – no symptoms, 5 – severe symptoms)

Yesterday I... ....
(which may be affecting my symptoms today)

My waistline (bloating) is   UP   DOWN   THE SAME

Notes (including optional weigh-in) ....

Evening

Today's food:

Morning ....
....

Lunch ....
....

Evening ....

My tummy feels... ....

I would score my gut health as   0   1   2   3   4   5
(0 – no symptoms, 5 – severe symptoms)

Opportunities for improvement..
....

Wins ....

DAY 19: INTRODUCING GASSY VEG 1 ....

Morning

Last night I slept... ....
....

This morning I feel... ....

My tummy feels... ....

I would score my gut health as   0   1   2   3   4   5
(0 – no symptoms, 5 – severe symptoms)

Yesterday I... ....
(which may be affecting my symptoms today)

My waistline (bloating) is   UP   DOWN   THE SAME

Notes (including optional weigh-in) ....

Evening

Today's food:

    Morning   ....
                      ....

    Lunch   ....
                      ....

    Evening   ....

My tummy feels... ....

I would score my gut health as   0   1   2   3   4   5
(0 – no symptoms, 5 – severe symptoms)

Opportunities for improvement..
....

Wins   ....

DAY 20: INTRODUCING GASSY VEG 2

Morning

Last night I slept... ....

....

This morning I feel... ....

My tummy feels... ....

I would score my gut health as   0   1   2   3   4   5
(0 – no symptoms, 5 – severe symptoms)

Yesterday I... ....
(which may be affecting my symptoms today)

My waistline (bloating) is   UP   DOWN   THE SAME

Notes (including optional weigh-in) ....

Evening

Today's food:

   Morning   ....

                ....

   Lunch   ....

                ....

   Evening   ....

My tummy feels... ....

I would score my gut health as   0   1   2   3   4   5
(0 – no symptoms, 5 – severe symptoms)

Opportunities for improvement...

....

Wins   ....

DAY 21: INTRODUCING GASSY VEG 3 ....

Morning

Last night I slept… ....
....

This morning I feel… ....

My tummy feels… ....

I would score my gut health as   0   1   2   3   4   5
(0 – no symptoms, 5 – severe symptoms)

Yesterday I… ....
(which may be affecting my symptoms today)

My waistline (bloating) is   UP   DOWN   THE SAME

Notes (including optional weigh-in) ....

Evening

Today's food:

    Morning   ....
    ....

    Lunch   ....
    ....

    Evening   ....

My tummy feels… ....

I would score my gut health as   0   1   2   3   4   5
(0 – no symptoms, 5 – severe symptoms)

Opportunities for improvement...
....

Wins   ....

DAY 22: REST DAY OR ADVENTURE DAY

Morning

Last night I slept… ....

....

This morning I feel… ....

My tummy feels… ....

I would score my gut health as   0   1   2   3   4   5
(0 – no symptoms, 5 – severe symptoms)

Yesterday I… ....
(which may be affecting my symptoms today)

My waistline (bloating) is   UP   DOWN   THE SAME

Notes (including optional weigh-in) ....

Evening

Today's food:

    Morning ....

....

    Lunch ....

....

    Evening ....

My tummy feels… ....

I would score my gut health as   0   1   2   3   4   5
(0 – no symptoms, 5 – severe symptoms)

Opportunities for improvement..

....

Wins ....

DAY 23: INTRODUCING WHEAT 1 ....

Morning
Last night I slept... ....
....

This morning I feel... ....

My tummy feels... ....

I would score my gut health as   0   1   2   3   4   5
(0 – no symptoms, 5 – severe symptoms)

Yesterday I... ....
(which may be affecting my symptoms today)

My waistline (bloating) is   UP   DOWN   THE SAME

Notes (including optional weigh-in) ....

Evening
Today's food:

Morning   ....
....

Lunch   ....
....

Evening   ....

My tummy feels... ....

I would score my gut health as   0   1   2   3   4   5
(0 – no symptoms, 5 – severe symptoms)

Opportunities for improvement..
....

Wins ....

DAY 24: INTRODUCING WHEAT 2

Morning

Last night I slept… ....
....

This morning I feel… ....

My tummy feels… ....

I would score my gut health as   0   1   2   3   4   5
(0 – no symptoms, 5 – severe symptoms)

Yesterday I… ....
(which may be affecting my symptoms today)

My waistline (bloating) is   UP   DOWN   THE SAME

Notes (including optional weigh-in) ....

Evening

Today's food:

    Morning   ....
....

    Lunch   ....
....

    Evening   ....

My tummy feels… ....

I would score my gut health as   0   1   2   3   4   5
(0 – no symptoms, 5 – severe symptoms)

Opportunities for improvement...
....

Wins   ....

DAY 25: INTRODUCING WHEAT 3..

Morning

Last night I slept... ....

....

This morning I feel... ....

My tummy feels... ....

I would score my gut health as   0   1   2   3   4   5

(0 – no symptoms, 5 – severe symptoms)

Yesterday I... ....

(which may be affecting my symptoms today)

My waistline (bloating) is   UP   DOWN   THE SAME

Notes (including optional weigh-in) ....

Evening

Today's food:

Morning   ....

....

Lunch   ....

....

Evening   ....

My tummy feels... ....

I would score my gut health as   0   1   2   3   4   5

(0 – no symptoms, 5 – severe symptoms)

Opportunities for improvement...

....

Wins   ....

DAY 26: BETTER LIVING FOR YOU ....

Morning

Last night I slept... ....

....

This morning I feel... ....

My tummy feels... ....

I would score my gut health as   0   1   2   3   4   5
(0 – no symptoms, 5 – severe symptoms)

Yesterday I... ....
(which may be affecting my symptoms today)

My waistline (bloating) is   UP   DOWN   THE SAME

Notes (including optional weigh-in) ....

Evening

Today's food:

Morning ....

....

Lunch ....

....

Evening ....

My tummy feels... ....

I would score my gut health as   0   1   2   3   4   5
(0 – no symptoms, 5 – severe symptoms)

Opportunities for improvement...

....

Wins ....

DAY 27: BETTER LIVING FOR YOU ....

Morning

Last night I slept... ....
....

This morning I feel... ....

My tummy feels... ....

I would score my gut health as   0   1   2   3   4   5
(0 – no symptoms, 5 – severe symptoms)

Yesterday I... ....
(which may be affecting my symptoms today)

My waistline (bloating) is   UP   DOWN   THE SAME

Notes (including optional weigh-in) ....

Evening

Today's food:

    Morning   ....
....

    Lunch   ....
....

    Evening   ....

My tummy feels... ....

I would score my gut health as   0   1   2   3   4   5
(0 – no symptoms, 5 – severe symptoms)

Opportunities for improvement ....
....

Wins   ....

DAY 28: BETTER LIVING FOR YOU ....

Morning

Last night I slept... ....

....

This morning I feel... ....

My tummy feels... ....

I would score my gut health as   0   1   2   3   4   5
(0 – no symptoms, 5 – severe symptoms)

Yesterday I... ....
(which may be affecting my symptoms today)

My waistline (bloating) is   UP   DOWN   THE SAME

Notes (including optional weigh-in) ....

Evening

Today's food:

    Morning   ....

....

    Lunch   ....

....

    Evening   ....

My tummy feels... ....

I would score my gut health as   0   1   2   3   4   5
(0 – no symptoms, 5 – severe symptoms)

Opportunities for improvement...

....

Wins   ....

28-DAY REVIEW

You should complete the 28-Day Review during the **Better Living** phase. This is the final piece of the jigsaw that you take away with you at the end of the plan. You can see at a glance where your problem areas lie. Also, it's important to see how your overall gut health has changed during the programme. Note that the 28-Day Review can be found in a 'print out and keep' format from **http://www.52recipes.co.uk/28G/**

Milk Intolerance Score	....	SAFE	MILDLY INTOLERANT	INTOLERANT
Red Meat Intolerance Score	....	SAFE	MILDLY INTOLERANT	INTOLERANT
Nightshade Intolerance Score	....	SAFE	MILDLY INTOLERANT	INTOLERANT
Gassy Veg Intolerance Score	....	SAFE	MILDLY INTOLERANT	INTOLERANT
Wheat Intolerance Score	....	SAFE	MILDLY INTOLERANT	INTOLERANT

If you think back to before you started the plan, what is the biggest change you notice between then and now?

....

....

Is there a difference between your Initial Gut-Health Assessment and how you assess your gut health now?

....

....

What were your three biggest successes?

1 ....

2 ....

3 ....

Review your food-trigger intolerances and assess your progress. Did you notice any improvements? If you had any setbacks, how will you tackle them?

....

....

What was the biggest lesson you learned about your own personal gut health?

....

....

What do you feel grateful for?

....

....

BONUSES

As a special thank you for purchasing **The 28-Day Gut-Health Plan**, I've got some amazing bonuses to get you started:

Bonus 1: Safe and Gut-friendly Food List:
Print out and keep this list. Stick it on your fridge.

Bonus 2: Full 28-Day Gut-Health Diary and 28-Day Review:
I know it's easier to have your own printable copy instead of struggling to write in a paperback or e-book. One page per day. You can use it again and again.

Bonus 3: Bonus Gut-friendly Recipes:
Perfectly Gluten-free Flatbread and *Probiotic Balsamic Salad Dressing*

All these bonuses are ready and waiting for you here: http://www.52recipes.co.uk/28G/

Part 3

RECIPES

STEP UP RECIPES

These are recipes where you have options to add ingredients as the weeks progress. They introduce a small amount of a test food group each week. After that meal, if you have any symptoms this will help you to pinpoint your sensitivities. These recipes are a really important part of the programme; other recipes you can pick and choose, but these you should try if at all possible.

Firstly, the Step Up recipes don't contain any irritants, so are great 'safe' recipes that you can use time and time again during the Rest and Restore phase. If you have a setback, you know that you can go back to the recipes and reset.

Secondly, these recipes develop over the weeks, with 'test' ingredients for checking intolerance added one at a time. Knowing that the week one 'control' recipe is safe, if you have a reaction to any added ingredients you will learn that this may be a problem food for you.

Also included are three safe recipes – my core 'safe' foods. The bread and brownies can both be made and frozen individually so that you have something to reach for when hunger calls. The poached egg is just an amazingly simple recipe that I recommend for anyone that loves eggs! Obviously, you can also use the bread to 'Step Up' and have it with different toppings as part of your Introducing Phases.

CHIA CHOC GRANOLA

Serves 7 / Ready in 30 minutes

200g (7oz) jumbo oats
20g (¾oz) flaked almonds
20g (¾oz) chia seeds
2 tbsp (30ml) mild (light) olive oil
1 heaped tsp (10g/⅓oz) butter
1 heaped tbsp (40g/1½oz) maple syrup
40g (1½oz) dark chocolate chips

- Preheat the oven to 160°C/Fan 140°C /325°F/Gas mark 3. Line a baking tray with a deep lip with greaseproof (waxed) paper or a silicone sheet.

- In a large bowl, combine the oats, almonds and chia seeds.

- Place the olive oil, butter and maple syrup in a small non-stick saucepan. Heat very gently, stirring until the butter has melted and the ingredients have combined. Do not allow to bubble or boil.

- Remove from the heat and pour into the oat mix. Mix together until all the oats have a light coating of the sweet butter. When fully coated, tip out onto the prepared baking tray and distribute; allow some gaps and a few clumps to form on the tray rather than spreading evenly. Bake in the hot oven for 18–20 minutes.

- Remove from the oven and allow to cool completely on the tray. When cool, lightly break up larger pieces of granola. Sprinkle the chocolate chips over the top. Transfer to a lidded jar or airtight container and store until needed.

Chia Choc Granola (Safe Edition)

Serve with 100ml (3½ fl oz) lactose-free milk.

Chia Choc Granola (Dairy Edition)

Serve with 100ml (3½ fl oz) semi-skimmed milk or 100g (3½oz) natural yogurt.

Chia Choc Granola (Gluten Edition)

Simply replace the maple syrup in the recipe with malt extract. Note that malt extract is made from barley, so will contain barley gluten. It is, however, wheat-free.

THE RICE BOX LUNCH

Most of us are out and about at lunchtime, so don't have time to make something hot. It's oh-so-easy to reach for a shop-bought sandwich made with cheap bread and spread with mayo. This rice box lunch can be made in five minutes in the morning or the night before. It makes two portions and lasts forty-eight hours. To make it even easier I recommend pouches of pre-cooked rice, which save time and give you exactly the right amount of rice.

There are several options for the 'safe' salad plus opportunities to build and test for nightshade and gas-producing or 'gassy' vegetables.

Finally, there are a few precautions to take when cooking and cooling rice, as there is a small risk of food poisoning. You should cook the rice as per the pack instructions and then allow to cool before combining with the salad ingredients. Serve the rice from chilled and do not reheat.

Makes 2 portions / Ready in 5 minutes
250g (9oz) cooked and cooled basmati rice (brown or white)
40g (1½oz) baby leaf spinach
2 spring onions (scallions), green parts only, chopped
100g (3½oz) cucumber (about 5cm/2in), chopped

For the dressing:

2 tsp extra-virgin olive oil

2 basil leaves, torn (or ½ tsp dried Italian herbs)

1 tsp English mustard

2 tsp apple cider vinegar

1 tsp balsamic vinegar

salt and freshly ground black pepper

- Place the basmati rice in a large bowl and break up the grains with a fork. Add the spinach, green parts of the spring onions (scallions) and cucumber and stir together.

- In a small bowl or cup, combine the olive oil, basil, mustard, cider and balsamic vinegars and season generously with salt and pepper.

- Pour over the rice and mix together.

- Divide between 2 bowls or containers, then add the extra filling ingredients as required.

Rice Box Lunch (Safe Edition)

To the basic rice salad add any of the following:

100g (3½oz) tinned salmon

100g (3½oz) smoked salmon, cut into strips

120g (4oz) cooked chicken pieces

2 large hard-boiled eggs

60g (2oz) feta cheese, cubed

Rice Box Lunch (Nightshade Edition)

Add 10 cherry tomatoes to the salad, washed and halved.

Or add 6 piquante red peppers from a jar, halved, plus a teaspoon of their juice.

Rice Box Lunch (Gassy Veg Edition)

Use the whole of the spring onions (scallions), not just the green parts.

Replace the protein with a tin of haricot beans (navy) or butter beans (lima). Rinse and drain the beans before adding to the salad.

SENSITIVE BELLIES' CHICKEN KORMA

This mild and creamy curry sauce is so easy to make and can be combined with chicken, fish or 'safe' vegetables. A tin of coconut milk consists of a thick coconut cream (normally on the top) and coconut water. We only need the cream for this recipe. Both the curry leaves and asafoetida can be bought at the supermarket. Don't be tempted to leave ingredients out, as each is important for a 'real' curry flavour. Serve with basmati rice.

Serves 2 / Ready in 15 minutes
1 x 400g (14oz) tin coconut milk
2 curry leaves
½ tsp salt
1 tsp asafoetida
½ tsp ground coriander
1 thumb ginger, peeled and grated (with a fine grater)
1 spring onion (scallion) green part only, chopped
1 tsp garlic oil
2 x 125g (4oz) skinless chicken breast fillets, diced
juice of ½ lime
1 handful of fresh coriander, roughly chopped

● From a tin of coconut milk, scoop out the cream at the top and place in a medium saucepan. Reserve the coconut water for later use, adding a tablespoon at a time if the sauce is a little thick.

● Place the saucepan over a very low heat. Add the curry leaves, salt, asafoetida, ground coriander, grated ginger and the green part of the spring onion (scallion), and stir.

- After a few minutes the curry will start to steam. Remove from the heat and leave for at least 5 minutes for the flavours to develop. The sauce can be frozen at this stage if required.
- Heat the garlic oil in a frying pan (skillet) on a medium heat. Add the chicken and fry lightly for a couple of minutes on each side.
- Remove the curry leaves from the sauce and pour the curry sauce into the frying pan (skillet). Bring to a gentle simmer and cook for 8–10 minutes or until the chicken is just cooked.
- Take the curry off the heat and stir in the lime juice and fresh coriander. Serve immediately over basmati rice.

Using the base Chicken Korma recipe to test your intolerances

If you've tried the Chicken Korma recipe during the Rest and Restore phase, you're ready to try adding other ingredients to test for intolerances. You can use the Chicken Korma recipe to test for Nightshade (tomato), Gas-Producing, or gassy (onion) and Dairy (cream). You should only test one ingredient at a time.

Chicken Korma (Nightshade Edition)

Wash and roughly chop 2 medium tomatoes and add to the curry sauce with the ginger and (green) spring onion (scallion). Cook as normal. Make sure you note down any stomach disturbances you experience in the 2 hours after you eat, overnight and up to 24 hours later.

Chicken Korma (Gassy Edition)

There are two levels of adding onion to this dish. Start with the whole spring onion (scallion), rather than just the green part, and move up to a small white onion the next time.

Spring onion (scallion): trim and chop 2 spring onions (scallions), using both the white and green parts. Add to the curry sauce at the same time as the ginger.

White onion: do this INSTEAD of adding spring onion to the sauce. Peel and finely chop a small white onion. Fry the onion in the garlic oil for 2 minutes before adding the chicken, then cook as normal.

Note any stomach disturbances 2 hours after eating and when you wake up the next morning.

Chicken Korma (Dairy Edition)

Replace a quarter of the coconut cream with 50ml (2fl oz) of double (thick) cream.

Note any stomach disturbances and also look out for sinus pain and skin changes.

NO-FUSS 'SAFE' STOCK

Serves 2 (just multiply the quantities to make more portions) / Ready in 1¼ hours

1 carrot, peeled and chopped
2 celery sticks, trimmed and chopped
2 chicken drumsticks, skin on
1 litre (1¾ pints) boiling water
8 whole peppercorns
1 bay leaf
1 tsp salt

- Simply place the carrot, celery and chicken drumsticks in a large saucepan. Pour over the boiling water and heat to a gentle simmer.

- Add the peppercorns, bay leaf and salt.

- Simmer gently for 1 hour.

- Remove from the heat and strain the liquid through a sieve. Discard the chicken and veggies.

The stock can be kept for 2 days in the fridge, frozen or used immediately.

ONE-POT CHICKEN STEW

One of the difficulties facing someone who is trying to avoid certain foodstuffs is that ANY processed food can contain troublesome ingredients. To make a stew we would often use a stock cube (or even fresh stock from the supermarket) but these will ALL contain onion in some form or another. So this recipe starts with making a very simple 'no-fuss' stock that only takes an hour and a quarter. The stock uses very economical chicken drumsticks that are then discarded. We use the No-fuss 'Safe' Stock as the basis for the stew.

One-pot Chicken Stew (Safe Edition)

Serves 2 / Ready in 30 minutes

1 litre (1¾ pints) No-fuss 'Safe' Stock (see page 142)
200g (7oz) waxy potatoes, peeled and chopped
1 small parsnip, peeled and chopped
1 small carrot, peeled and chopped
1 tbsp tamari sauce
2 tsp English mustard
2 spring onions (scallions), green parts only, trimmed and finely chopped
a pinch of freshly ground black pepper
2 x 125g (4oz) skinless chicken breast fillets, halved

- Bring the stock to a simmer in a saucepan. Add the potatoes, parsnip and carrot. Simmer for 15 minutes.

- Add the tamari sauce, mustard, green spring onions (scallions), pepper and chicken pieces. Simmer for 10–12 minutes until the chicken is cooked through. Crush a few of the potatoes with the back of a fork and stir through to naturally thicken the sauce.

- Distribute the veggies between 2 plates or shallow bowls. Place the chicken pieces on top. Then pour over the remaining sauce.

One-pot Chicken Stew (Dairy Edition)

Add 2 tablespoons double (thick) cream just before serving.

One-pot Chicken Stew (Gassy Veg Edition)

Add 1 x 400g (14oz) tin butter beans (lima beans), rinsed and drained. Add the beans at the same time as the chicken. You can also use the white part of the spring onion (scallion).

TUMMY-FRIENDLY RED PASTA SAUCE

Pasta and tomato sauce can be one of the worst meals for sensitive tums. There's gluten in the pasta, plus onions, garlic, tomatoes … This tomato-free sauce uses every trick in the book to make a delicious sauce that looks and tastes like a real tomato sauce. Serve with a gluten-free pasta such as buckwheat.

Serves 4 / Ready in 30 minutes

250g (9oz) cooked beetroot, chopped into chunks
4 carrots, peeled and chopped
1 tbsp garlic oil
1 handful of fresh basil, stalks and leaves separated
250ml (9fl oz) No-fuss 'Safe' Stock (see page 142)
1 tsp salt
1 tsp dried oregano
1 tsp asafoetida
2 tsp capers
1 tsp lemon juice

- Place the beetroot and carrots in a saucepan of boiling water and simmer for 15 minutes. Drain and set aside.
- Heat the garlic oil on a low heat and add the beetroot and carrots. Chop the basil stalks finely and add to the pan. Fry gently for 5 minutes.
- Add the stock, salt, oregano and asafoetida and simmer for 10 minutes. Remove from the heat and stir in the basil leaves, capers and lemon juice. Transfer to a food processor and blend. You can leave it a little chunky or go for a very smooth sauce. The sauce can be chilled or frozen at this stage.
- Heat in a small pan on the hob for 5 minutes before serving.

Red Pasta Sauce (Nightshade Edition)

Replace the stock with a tin of chopped tomatoes. You could also add some chopped red pepper and/or a teaspoon of chilli flakes.

Red Pasta Sauce (Red Meat Edition)

Fry 3 slices of bacon (chopped) and add to the blitzed sauce.

If you want to serve this as a bolognese-style sauce, then fry 500g (18oz) minced beef until browned, add the blitzed sauce and cook for 30–45 minutes over a low heat.

Red Pasta Sauce (Gassy Veg Edition)

Fry chopped onion and garlic with the beetroot and carrot. Use normal olive oil in place of the garlic oil.

SEEDED GLUTEN-FREE BREAD

Gluten-free bread isn't the same as real bread. It's denser, looks less appealing and rises less. Yet, I've found having a bread alternative available gives you so many more options. I like this mix (which I have perfected over many attempts) as I think it balances out all the tastes to be as good as gluten-free bread can be. And it's much better than shop-bought gluten-free. As with all gluten-free breads, this tastes best still warm and fresh, or toasted.

The best way to use and store this bread is to wait until it's completely cool, and cut into thin slices. Freeze the bread and bring out and toast individual slices when you need them.

Makes 12 slices / Ready in 1½ hours

400ml (14fl oz) water
1 tsp apple cider vinegar
3 tbsp mild (light) olive oil
400g (14oz) brown gluten-free bread flour
1 tbsp sugar
1 tsp salt
50g (2oz) buckwheat flour
1 tsp psyllium husks
2 tsp yeast
1 tbsp sesame seeds
2 tbsp pumpkin seeds

In a bread machine:

- Put the water, vinegar and mild (light) olive oil in the base of the bread pan. Add the gluten-free flour on top of the liquid and then the sugar and salt.
- In a separate bowl or jar, mix together the buckwheat flour and psyllium husks; psyllium goes all lumpy if it's not mixed into another flour before adding to water. Add to the pan.
- Finally, add the yeast, sesame seeds and pumpkin seeds.
- Bake on the gluten-free setting with a 'dark crust' in your bread maker.

By hand:

- In a jug, mix together the water, vinegar and olive oil.
- Thoroughly mix together the two flours, sugar, salt, psyllium, yeast, sesame and pumpkin seeds in a large bowl. Pour the liquid into the flour and yeast mixture and stir slowly. Finally, bring together with your hands to make a dough.

- Tip the dough into an oiled and lined 1kg (2lb) bread tin. Cover with cling film and leave to rise for 25 minutes.
- Preheat the oven to 220°C/Fan 200°C/425°F/Gas mark 7.
- Bake for 55–60 minutes.

AMAZING 'ONE-MINUTE' MICROWAVE POACHED EGG

This is my go-to emergency recipe for any time of day. I serve it on a slice of gluten-free toast. It makes everything all right in the world.

Serves 1 / Ready in 1 minute
½ tsp white wine vinegar
125ml (4½fl oz) water
1 large egg, straight from the fridge

- Take a small microwave-safe bowl or cup. A ramekin or similar would work well.
- Put the vinegar in the bottom of the bowl and swirl round. Tip the excess away, then fill the bowl to about two-thirds full of water. Crack the egg on the edge of the dish and hold near the water as you gently plop it into the bowl. Cover loosely with cling film.
- Carry gently to the microwave. Microwave for 1 minute. Remove from the water with a dessertspoon. Perfect poached egg every time.

SALTED OLIVE OIL BROWNIES

Everyone needs a treat and these soft, fudgy brownies are mine! Yes, they contain sugar – I don't see how you can bake properly without it. But there's so much good stuff here. I love olive oil and the extra-virgin olive oil in these brownies gives it a delicate, fruity taste. Allow yourself one every now and again as a reward for cutting out other things, knowing that these are so much better for you than anything shop-bought.

Makes 12 brownies / Ready in 45 minutes
90g (3oz) caster (fine) sugar
90g (3oz) dark brown sugar
120ml (4fl oz) extra-virgin olive oil, plus extra for oiling
200g (7oz) 70% dark chocolate
3 eggs, beaten
1 tsp vanilla essence
zest of ½ lime
80g ground almonds
1 tsp psyllium husks
a pinch of salt
flaky sea salt, for sprinkling

- Preheat the oven to 180°C/Fan 160°C/350°F/Gas mark 4. Grease with olive oil and line the bottom of a 20cm (8in) springform round cake tin or similar-sized square tin with baking parchment.

- Combine the two types of sugar in a large bowl.

- In a small saucepan, heat the olive oil over a very low heat. Break in the chocolate and stir until it starts to melt. Remove from the heat and continue stirring until all the chocolate has melted into the oil.

- Pour the chocolate into the sugars and beat well. Add the beaten eggs a little at a time, mixing well after each addition. Stir in the vanilla and lime zest.

- In a separate bowl, thoroughly combine the ground almonds, psyllium husks and salt. Pour in the chocolate mixture and mix until just combined.

- Pour the batter into the cake tin and bake for 30–40 minutes. Allow to cool in the tin for 10 minutes before carefully removing to a wire rack. Sprinkle with the sea salt. When fully cool, cut into 12 pieces and store in an airtight container. These brownies can also be frozen.

REST AND RESTORE RECIPES

TWO-INGREDIENT BANANA PANCAKES

Wheat & Gluten Free ✓	Lactose Free ✓	Nightshade Free ✓
Gassy Veg Free ✓	Red Meat Free ✓	

Serves 1 / Ready in 5 minutes

1 banana

2 eggs

1 tsp mild (light) olive oil

- Use the back of a fork to thoroughly mash the banana.

- In a separate bowl, whisk the eggs. Add the banana to the whisked eggs.

- Heat the oil in a medium frying pan (skillet) until hot but not smoking. Pour in the pancake mix. Cook for 3–4 minutes, turning if you dare, until just cooked but still a little wobbly.

EASY MICROWAVE PORRIDGE

Wheat & Gluten Free ✓	Lactose Free ✓	Nightshade Free ✓
Gassy Veg Free ✓	Red Meat Free ✓	

Serves 1 / Ready in 3 minutes

40g (1½oz) porridge oats (oatmeal)

100ml (3½fl oz) lacto free milk

120ml (4fl oz) water

- Simply combine the oats, milk and water in a high-sided microwave-safe bowl or jug.

- Microwave on high power for 2 minutes, stir thoroughly, then microwave for a further minute. Stir again and add a little extra milk, if necessary, to gain the right consistency.

HONEY POPCORN CEREAL

Wheat & Gluten Free ✓	Lactose Free ✓	Nightshade Free ✓
Gassy Veg Free ✓	Red Meat Free ✓	

Serves 4 / Ready in 25 minutes

1 tbsp mild (light) olive oil
1 tbsp (15g/½oz) butter
1 tbsp honey
¼ tsp cinnamon
100g (3½oz) popped corn
30g (1oz) peanuts, chopped
lactose-free milk, to serve

- Preheat the oven to 150°C/Fan 130°C /300°F/Gas mark 2.
- Place the olive oil, butter, honey and cinnamon in a small pan. Heat together until the butter has melted and the ingredients have combined.
- Put the popped corn and peanuts in a large bowl and pour over the honey mixture. Stir well to give a light, even coating.
- Tip the popcorn onto a baking tray, scooping up any mixture from the bottom of the bowl and drizzling it over. Bake for 20 minutes.
- Remove from the oven and allow to cool completely on the tray before transferring to an airtight container.
- Serve with lactose-free milk.

CACAO SNACK POT CEREAL

Wheat & Gluten Free ✓	Lactose Free ✓	Nightshade Free ✓
Gassy Veg Free ✓	Red Meat Free ✓	

Serves 4 / Ready in 1 minute

25g (1oz) cacao nibs
80g (3oz) chopped dates

- Simply combine the nibs and dates and store in an airtight jar until needed.
- To eat it as a cereal, combine with some jumbo oats and serve with lactose-free milk.

LEMON PEPPER CHICKEN

Wheat & Gluten Free ✓	Lactose Free ✓	Nightshade Free ✓
Gassy Veg Free ✓	Red Meat Free ✓	

Serves 2 / Ready in 15 minutes

2 skinless chicken breast fillets (about 125g/4oz each)

1 tbsp olive oil

zest of 1 lemon

½ tsp dried thyme

juice of 2 lemons

1 tsp sugar

250g (9oz) pre-cooked brown basmati rice

salt and freshly ground black pepper

- Cut the chicken breasts in half widthways, making 2 fat pieces. Use a meat tenderizer (or rolling pin covered in cling film) to bash the chicken pieces until they are no more than 1cm/½in thick.

- Heat the oil in a frying pan (skillet) over a medium–high heat. When hot, add the chicken pieces. Sprinkle over the lemon zest and thyme and season generously with black pepper. Cook the pieces for about 2 minutes each side, until golden and just cooked through, so the juices run clear when cut.

- Add the lemon juice to the pan, together with the sugar and a pinch of salt. Reduce the heat to low and allow the sauce to bubble around the chicken for 2 minutes. Transfer the chicken to a warm plate using a slotted spoon.

- Add the rice to the pan and stir into the sauce, separating any clumps. Cook for 3–4 minutes until the rice is hot and all the sauce has been absorbed. Distribute the rice between 2 plates and place the chicken on the top.

DELICATE THAI CHICKEN CURRY

Wheat & Gluten Free ✓	Lactose Free ✓	Nightshade Free ✓
Gassy Veg Free ✓	Red Meat Free ✓	

Serves 2 / Ready in 15 minutes

1 tsp sesame oil

2 skinless chicken breast fillets (each about 125g/4oz), cut into pieces

2 spring onions (scallions), green parts only, chopped

1 thumb ginger, peeled and finely grated

1 tsp lemongrass paste

1 tsp galangal paste

zest and juice of 1 lime

1 x 400g (14oz) tin light coconut milk, cream only

4 basil leaves, finely chopped

1 small handful of coriander (cilantro), finely chopped

1 tsp brown sugar

1 tbsp fish sauce

1 small handful of coriander (cilantro), to serve

- Heat the sesame oil in a large frying pan (skillet) or wok. Add the chicken and cook for 3–4 minutes each side until browned all over.

- Add the green part of the spring onions (scallions), ginger, lemongrass paste, galangal paste and lime zest. Stir-fry for 1 minute. Scoop the cream off the top of the can of coconut milk and add to the pan. Reserve the coconut water to add a little later if the curry is too thick.

- Over a medium heat, warm the curry until it is gently simmering. Add the basil, coriander (cilantro), brown sugar, fish sauce and lime juice. Simmer for 4 minutes.

- Serve with the remaining coriander (cilantro) sprinkled over.

QUICK FETA BURGERS

Wheat & Gluten Free ✓	Lactose Free ✓	Nightshade Free ✓
Gassy Veg Free ✓	Red Meat Free ✓	

Serves 2 / Ready in 15 minutes

2 courgettes (zucchini), trimmed

2 spring onions (scallions), green parts only, finely chopped

100g (3½oz) feta cheese, crumbled

1 small handful of fresh parsley, chopped

1 tsp asafoetida

1 level tbsp buckwheat (or other gluten-free) flour

1 large egg, beaten

1 tbsp olive oil

salt and freshly ground black pepper

- Coarsely grate the courgettes (zucchini) and lay out on kitchen paper (paper towels) to dry out. Leave for about 10 minutes, then pat the top of the courgettes to get rid of any extra moisture.

- Mix the green part of the spring onions (scallions), crumbled feta, parsley and asafoetida in a large bowl. Season with salt and pepper and stir in the flour. Pour in the beaten egg and mix well. Finally, mix in the grated courgettes.

- Heat the oil in a wide frying pan (skillet) over a medium–high heat. When hot, add tablespoon-sized scoops of the mixture to the pan, flattening each scoop with the back of the spoon as you go. The burgers need to be widely spaced so you may have to do this in 2 batches. Fry for about 2 minutes on each side until golden. Serve immediately.

'THOUSAND ISLAND' CHICKEN SALAD

Wheat & Gluten Free ✓	Lactose Free ✓	Nightshade Free ✓
Gassy Veg Free ✓	Red Meat Free ✓	

Serves 2 / Ready in 5 minutes

2 heaped tbsp light mayonnaise

1 tsp dried chives

2 tsp red wine vinegar

½ tsp Dijon mustard

a few drops of Worcestershire sauce

¼ tsp asafoetida

½ iceberg lettuce (200g), chopped

10cm(4in) piece cucumber, diced

250g (9oz) cooked chicken, sliced

freshly ground black pepper

- Mix together the mayonnaise, chives, vinegar, mustard, Worcestershire sauce, asafoetida and a little black pepper. Leave to rest for at least 5 minutes. (It tastes even better if refrigerated for a few hours.)

- Place the lettuce and cucumber in a large bowl and pour two-thirds of the dressing over. If the dressing is a little thick, add a few drops of water to thin. Mix the dressing into the salad. Divide between 2 plates. Top with the sliced chicken and drizzle over the rest of the dressing.

SMOKED SALMON KEDGEREE

Wheat & Gluten Free ✓	Lactose Free ✓	Nightshade Free ✓
Gassy Veg Free ✓	Red Meat Free ✓	

Serves 2 / Ready in 15 minutes

1 tbsp butter

1 cardamom pod, split with the back of a spoon

½ tsp asafoetida

¼ tsp cinnamon

½ tsp turmeric

1 bay leaf

150g (5oz) uncooked basmati rice

350ml (12fl oz) No-fuss 'Safe' Stock (see page 142)

1 large egg, at room temp

1 small handful of fresh parsley, chopped

250g (9oz) smoked salmon, cut into thick strips

salt and freshly ground black pepper

- Melt the butter in a large, lidded saucepan. Add the cardamom, asafoetida, cinnamon, turmeric and bay leaf. Season with salt and pepper.

- Tip in the rice and toss through until each grain is coated in the butter. Add the stock and bring to the boil. Stir once, then put the lid on the pan and turn the heat to low. Cook gently for 12 minutes.

- Meanwhile, boil the egg for 8 minutes, then transfer to cold water to cool. Peel and quarter.

- Uncover the rice and remove the cardamom and bay leaf. Stir through the parsley.

- Transfer the rice to a serving dish or 2 plates. Arrange the smoked salmon and egg over the top.

HONG KONG PRAWNS

Wheat & Gluten Free ✓	Lactose Free ✓	Nightshade Free ✓
Gassy Veg Free ✓	Red Meat Free ✓	

Serves 2 / Ready in 10 minutes

250g (9oz) raw king prawns (king or jumbo shrimp)

zest and juice of 1 lime

1 tsp fish sauce

½ tsp sugar

1 tsp olive oil

200g (7oz) green beans, trimmed

1 spring onion (scallion), green part only, trimmed and finely chopped

1 handful of fresh coriander (cilantro), chopped

30g (1oz) salted peanuts, roughly chopped or bashed

salt and freshly ground black pepper

- Dry the prawns (shrimp) with kitchen paper (paper towels) and season with salt and pepper.

- Put the zest of the lime into a small bowl and half the lime juice. Stir in the fish sauce and sugar.

- Heat the oil in a wide frying pan (skillet) over a medium–high heat. When the oil is hot, add the prawns, green beans and the green part of the spring onion (scallion). Stir-fry for 3 minutes. Reduce the heat and stir in the fish sauce mixture. Cook for 1 more minute or until the prawns are cooked through.

- Turn off the heat and toss through the coriander (cilantro) and peanuts. Serve immediately with the remaining lime juice drizzled over.

CHICKEN IN WHITE WINE

Wheat & Gluten Free ✓	Lactose Free ✓	Nightshade Free ✓
Gassy Veg Free ✓	Red Meat Free ✓	

Serves 2 / Ready in 15 minutes

1 tsp garlic oil

2 spring onions (scallions), green parts only, trimmed and sliced

1 carrot, peeled and finely diced

½ tsp dried mixed herbs

2 × 150g (5oz) skinless chicken breast fillets, both halved

150g (5oz) green beans, trimmed

200ml (7fl oz) dry white wine

1 tsp cornflour (cornstarch), mixed with a little cold water to make a paste

1 heaped tsp butter

1 handful of fresh parsley, chopped

- Heat the garlic oil, green part of the spring onions (scallions), carrot and dried mixed herbs in a small, lidded frying pan (skillet) or saucepan for 1–2 minutes until sizzling. Add the chicken and cook for about 4 minutes until the first side turns golden.

- Turn the chicken over and add the green beans and white wine. Put the lid on and as soon as it starts to simmer, turn the heat to low. Allow the chicken to continue to cook in the wine for a further 5 minutes. Check that the meat is cooked through before removing the chicken and beans from the pan with a slotted spoon and covering.

- Bring the remaining liquid in the pan back up to simmering and stir in the cornflour (cornstarch) and butter. Bubble for 2 minutes while the sauce thickens a little. Stir in the parsley.

- Arrange the chicken on the plate and then add the sauce.

OVEN-BAKED SWEET POTATO WEDGES

Wheat & Gluten Free ✓	Lactose Free ✓	Nightshade Free ✓
Gassy Veg Free ✓	Red Meat Free ✓	

Serves 2 / Ready in 45 minutes

2 sweet potatoes

1 tbsp olive oil

salt and freshly ground black pepper

- Preheat the oven to 220°C/Fan 200°C/425°F/Gas mark 7.

- Peel and cut the sweet potatoes into large wedges. If you prefer, you can leave the skin on the potatoes.

- Place the sweet potato wedges into a pan of cold, salted water and bring to the boil. Cook for 15 minutes. Drain and leave to cool until they are cold enough to handle.

- Place the sweet potatoes in a roasting tray and pour on the oil. Toss through with your hands so that the potatoes are as well covered as possible and season well.

- Bake in the oven for 25–30 minutes until crispy and golden.

MANGO CURRY WITH PRAWNS

Wheat & Gluten Free ✓	Lactose Free ✓	Nightshade Free ✓
Gassy Veg Free ✓	Red Meat Free ✓	

Serves 2 / Ready in 20–25 minutes

1 x 400g (14oz) tin light coconut milk

1 tsp asafoetida

1 heaped tsp lemongrass paste

1 large thumb (5cm/2in) ginger, peeled and grated

4 basil leaves, finely chopped

2 tbsp fish sauce

zest and juice of 1 lime

200g mango, cut into chunks (frozen is fine)

250g raw king prawns (king or jumbo shrimp)

1 large handful of fresh coriander (cilantro), roughly chopped

- Heat the coconut milk in a frying pan (skillet) or wok over a high heat. Bring to the boil, then simmer for 10–15 minutes until reduced.

- Meanwhile, combine the asafoetida, lemongrass paste, ginger, basil, fish sauce and lime zest and juice in a small bowl. Tip into the reduced coconut milk and simmer for 4 minutes.

- Add the mango and king prawns (shrimp). Bring back to a simmer and cook for 3–4 minutes until the prawns are pink and cooked through. Stir through the coriander (cilantro) just before serving.

WARM CHICKEN SALAD

Wheat & Gluten Free ✓	Lactose Free ✓	Nightshade Free ✓
Gassy Veg Free ✓	Red Meat Free ✓	

Serves 2 / Ready in 35 minutes

300g (11oz) butternut squash, cut into wedges
2 x 125g/4oz chicken breasts (skin on)
1 tbsp olive oil
1 stalk fresh rosemary or 1 tsp dried
salt and freshly ground black pepper
80g (3oz) rocket (arugula)

For the dressing:
juice of ½ lemon
1 tsp extra-virgin olive oil
1 tsp white wine vinegar
1 tsp maple syrup
½ tsp Dijon mustard

- Preheat the oven to 220°C/Fan 200°C/425°F/Gas mark 7.

- In a large bowl, toss together the butternut squash, chicken breasts, olive oil, rosemary and salt and pepper. Place the chicken breasts on a baking tray (skin-side up) and arrange the butternut squash around them. Bake for 25 minutes. Check that the chicken is fully cooked before serving, so that the juices run clear when cut.

- Remove the skin from the chicken breasts and cut into fat strips.

- To make the dressing, whisk together the lemon juice, extra-virgin olive oil, vinegar, maple syrup and Dijon mustard.

- Place the rocket (arugula) in a large bowl and toss through the dressing. Add the butternut squash and chicken. Serve warm.

TERIYAKI-GLAZED SALMON WITH STIR-FRIED RICE NOODLES

Wheat & Gluten Free ✓	Lactose Free ✓	Nightshade Free ✓
Gassy Veg Free ✓	Red Meat Free ✓	

Serves 2 / Ready in 20 minutes

1 tbsp tamari sauce

1 tbsp water

1 tsp cornflour (cornstarch)

1 tbsp honey

1 tbsp rice vinegar

½ tsp ground ginger

2 salmon fillets (skin on)

1 tsp sesame oil

1 carrot, peeled and julienned

100g (3½oz) baby corn

200g (7oz) rice noodles, cooked

1 lime, quartered, to serve

- Whisk together the tamari sauce, water, cornflour (cornstarch), honey, rice vinegar and ground ginger. Heat in a small pan until thickened, stirring continuously. Pour over the salmon and leave to marinate for 5 minutes.

- Heat the sesame oil in a frying pan (skillet) over a medium–high heat. Add the salmon skin-side down and lower the heat to medium. Cook the salmon on one side for 5–6 minutes, then turn and add the carrot and baby corn. Cook for another 5–6 minutes until the salmon is cooked through. Remove the salmon from the pan and set aside.

- Add the rice noodles, the remaining teriyaki marinade and a little water. Stir-fry for a further 2 minutes.

- Divide the noodles between 2 plates and top with the salmon fillets. Squeeze over a little lime juice and serve with lime wedges on the side.

QUINOA AND BEETROOT SALAD WITH TAHINI

Wheat & Gluten Free ✓	Lactose Free ✓	Nightshade Free ✓
Gassy Veg Free ✓	Red Meat Free ✓	

Serves 2 / Ready in 20 minutes
For the dressing:
1 tsp extra-virgin olive oil
1 tsp apple cider vinegar
1 tsp balsamic vinegar
½ tsp English mustard
salt and freshly ground black pepper

For the tahini sauce:
1 heaped tbsp tahini paste
juice of ½ lemon
2 tsp garlic oil
a pinch of salt
a little water to thin, if necessary

For the salad:
80g (3oz) (dried weight) quinoa
150g (5oz) cooked beetroot, chopped
60g (2oz) young spinach leaves
1 spring onion (scallion), green part only, chopped

- Cook the quinoa in boiling water for about 15 minutes until tender.

- Make the dressing by whisking together the olive oil, cider vinegar, balsamic vinegar, mustard and salt and pepper.

- Make the tahini sauce by mixing together the tahini paste, lemon juice, garlic oil and a little salt. If it's too thick, add a little water.

- When the quinoa is cooked and cooled, transfer to a large bowl and add the beetroot, spinach leaves and green part of the spring onion. Stir together gently. Pour in the dressing and mix again. Distribute between 2 bowls (or use lunchbox containers – it's a great portable meal).
- Serve with the tahini on the side.

SALMON AND GINGER FISHCAKES

Wheat & Gluten Free ✓	Lactose Free ✓	Nightshade Free ✓
Gassy Veg Free ✓	Red Meat Free ✓	

Serves 2 / Ready in 30–50 minutes
1 x 200g (7oz) tin salmon, drained
a few chives, finely chopped
1 thumb ginger, peeled and grated
zest of 1 lime
1 tsp cornflour (cornstarch)
1 tsp olive oil, plus extra for oiling
salt and freshly ground black pepper

- Preheat the oven to 220°C/Fan 200°C/425°F/Gas mark 7. Lightly oil a baking tray.
- Flake the salmon into a bowl. Stir in the chives, ginger, lime zest, cornflour (cornstarch) and olive oil. Season with salt and pepper. Scoop out golf-ball-sized heaps of the mixture and gently press into shape with your hands. Place on the baking tray. Flatten the balls a little with the palm of your hand.
- Freeze for 10 minutes or refrigerate for 30 minutes to help the fishcakes keep their shape (optional).
- Bake for 15–18 minutes until tinged brown at the edges.

CARIBBEAN CHICKEN

Wheat & Gluten Free ✓	Lactose Free ✓	Nightshade Free ✓
Gassy Veg Free ✓	Red Meat Free ✓	

Serves 2 / Ready in 45 minutes (including 30 minutes marinating)

200g (7oz) skinless chicken breast fillet, cut into strips

25g (1oz) mango pieces, pulped with a fork

1 tbsp rum

juice of 1 lime

1 heaped tbsp desiccated (dry unsweetened) coconut

1 tbsp cornflour (cornstarch)

1 tbsp mild (light) olive oil

salt and freshly ground black pepper

- Place the chicken strips in a freezer bag. Add the mango, rum and lime juice. Press the air out of the bag and seal. Rub the marinade around the chicken and leave to rest in the fridge for 30 minutes to 1 hour.

- Preheat the oven to 200°C/Fan 180°C/400°F/Gas mark 6.

- Mix together the coconut and cornflour (cornstarch) with a little salt and pepper. Remove 1 strip of chicken at a time from the bag and toss in the coconut and flour mixture. Repeat with each piece of chicken.

- Take a wide frying pan, add the oil and set the heat to medium–high. Add the chicken pieces to the frying pan (skillet) one at a time, trying to leave room between the pieces. Fry for 2 minutes, until golden brown on one side, then turn and fry the other side for 2 minutes.

- Transfer the chicken pieces to a baking tray and bake in the oven for 10 minutes, or until cooked through, so that the juices run clear when cut.

POACHED SALMON SALAD

Wheat & Gluten Free ✓	Lactose Free ✓	Nightshade Free ✓
Gassy Veg Free ✓	Red Meat Free ✓	

Serves 1 / Ready in 15 minutes

1 salmon fillet (about 125g/5oz), skinless and boneless

½ lemon

1 bay leaf

a few peppercorns

60g (2oz) mixed salad leaves

30g (1oz) rocket (arugula) leaves

2 radishes, trimmed and sliced

100g (3½oz) cucumber (about 5cm/2in), cut into chunks

1 spring onion (scallion), green part only, sliced

For the dressing:

2 tsp light mayonnaise

1 tbsp rice wine vinegar

2 mint leaves, finely chopped

salt and freshly ground black pepper

- Place the salmon in a big enough pan for it to lie flat. Pour in boiling water until the salmon is just covered. Add lemon, bay leaf and peppercorns. Bring to a gentle simmer and cook for 10–12 minutes until the salmon is cooked. Remove from the pan with a slotted spoon and set aside to cool.

- To make the dressing, in a small bowl mix together the mayonnaise, rice wine vinegar, mint leaves and salt and pepper. Leave to stand for 5 minutes to allow the flavours to develop.

- Arrange the salad leaves and rocket (arugula) on a serving plate and top with the radishes, cucumber and green part of the spring onion (scallion).

- Flake the salmon onto the salad and drizzle the dressing over the top.

MUSHROOM RISOTTO

Wheat & Gluten Free ✓	Lactose Free ✓	Nightshade Free ✓
Gassy Veg Free ✓	Red Meat Free ✓	

Serves 2 / Ready in 30 minutes, plus 20 minutes soaking

25g (1oz) dried porcini mushrooms

500ml (18fl oz) boiling water

1 tbsp garlic oil

250g (9oz) chestnut mushrooms, washed and sliced

150g (5oz) arborio rice

175ml (6fl oz) white wine

500ml (18fl oz) No-fuss 'Safe' Stock (see page 142)

25g (1oz) butter

30g (1oz) Parmesan, finely grated

salt and freshly ground black pepper

- Put the porcini mushrooms in a bowl or jug and pour over the boiling water. Leave to soak for 20 minutes. Remove the mushrooms, squeezing any excess liquid back into the bowl. Chop the mushrooms. Reserve the liquid to use as a stock, discarding the dregs of the stock, which are grainy.

- Heat the garlic oil on a medium heat in a wide shallow pan. Stir in the fresh chestnut and dried porcini mushrooms. Season with salt and pepper. Heat for 7–8 minutes until the mushrooms are glossy and softened.

- Add the rice to the pan and stir through so that the oil covers every grain. Add the white wine and let it bubble away to next to nothing. Pour in half the mushroom stock, and keeping the pan on a medium heat cook until the rice has absorbed the liquid. Stir frequently. Add the rest of the mushroom stock.

- Cook until this stock is absorbed. Then add half the 'Safe' stock, and continue to simmer and stir. It should start to become creamy and plump. When all the stock has been absorbed, check that the rice is cooked. If it needs a little longer add a little bit more water.

- Take the pan off the heat and add the butter and half the Parmesan. Stir through and cover. Leave for 5 minutes for the last of the liquid to be absorbed. Give the risotto a final stir and serve with the remaining Parmesan sprinkled over.

BARBECUE CHICKEN WINGS

Wheat & Gluten Free ✓	Lactose Free ✓	Nightshade Free ✓
Gassy Veg Free ✓	Red Meat Free ✓	

Serves 4 / Ready in 35 minutes

1 heaped tsp dark brown sugar

½ tsp asafoetida

1 tsp dried oregano

1 tsp Dijon mustard

1 tbsp maple syrup

1 tsp cornflour (cornstarch), blended with a little water to form a paste

½ tsp Worcestershire sauce

1 tsp apple cider vinegar

a pinch of salt

2 tbsp water

1kg (2.2lb) chicken wings

- In a small bowl, combine the brown sugar, asafoetida, oregano, mustard, maple syrup, cornflour (cornstarch) paste, Worcestershire sauce, apple cider vinegar and pinch of salt. Slowly stir in a little water at a time until the sauce has the consistency of natural yogurt.

- Place the chicken wings in a large bowl and pour half the sauce over. Mix together with your hands until all the chicken wings are coated and cook either in the oven or on the grill (broiler) or barbecue (see below).

In the oven

Bake in an oven preheated to 190°C/Fan 170°C/375°F/Gas mark 5 for 25 minutes.

On the grill (broiler) or barbecue

Cook for 10–12 minutes each side on a medium heat.

When the chicken wings are cooked, pour over the rest of the sauce, rubbing a little into each wing with the back of a spoon.

EGG-FRIED RICE AND PRAWNS

Wheat & Gluten Free ✓	Lactose Free ✓	Nightshade Free ✓
Gassy Veg Free ✓	Red Meat Free ✓	

Serves 2 / Ready in 15 minutes

1 egg

1 tsp sesame oil

1 tbsp mild (light) olive oil

250g (7oz) cooked basmati rice

60g (2oz) green beans, trimmed

60g (2oz) baby corn

2 spring onions (scallions), green parts only, chopped

250g (9oz) raw king prawns (king or jumbo shrimp)

½ tsp white pepper

1 tsp tamari sauce

- Beat together the egg and sesame oil and set aside.

- Heat the olive oil in a wok or large frying pan (skillet) on a medium–high heat. When it's hot, add the rice and stir-fry for 3 minutes, breaking up any clumps of rice with the back of the spoon and making sure each grain is individually coated.

- Add the green beans, baby corn and prawns (shrimp). Stir-fry, turning the rice constantly around the pan, until the prawns are pink. Add the white pepper and tamari sauce, stir, then push to the side of the pan.

- Pour the beaten egg mixture into the other side of the pan and leave until it just begins to set. Swirl the egg around to break it up, then toss it through the rice.

BANANA KETCHUP

Wheat & Gluten Free ✓	Lactose Free ✓	Nightshade Free ✓
Gassy Veg Free ✓	Red Meat Free ✓	

Makes 1 jar / Ready in 20 minutes

1 tsp garlic oil

1 large thumb (5cm/2in) ginger, peeled and finely grated, mixed with 1 tablespoon water

½ tsp asafoetida

¼ tsp turmeric

¼ tsp ground allspice

½ tsp salt

2 large ripe bananas, thoroughly mashed

1 tbsp apple cider vinegar

1 tbsp honey

1 tbsp rum

1 tbsp tamari sauce

- Heat the garlic oil in a saucepan over a medium heat. Add the ginger, asafoetida, turmeric, allspice and salt. Stir-fry for a minute, until the ginger has soaked up the oil.

- Add the mashed bananas, vinegar, honey, rum and tamari sauce. Reduce the heat to low, cover, and cook for 15 minutes, stirring often. Remove from the heat and allow to cool.

- Thin with a little water if needed, then transfer to an airtight container and keep in the refrigerator for up to 2 weeks.

GLUTEN-FREE FLATBREAD

Wheat & Gluten Free ✓	Lactose Free ✓	Nightshade Free ✓
Gassy Veg Free ✓	Red Meat Free ✓	

Makes 6 flatbreads / Ready in 1 hour 15 minutes

100g (3½oz) ground almonds

25g (1oz) psyllium husks

2 tsp baking powder

½ tsp salt

250ml (9fl oz) boiling water

2 tsp apple cider vinegar

2 egg whites (at room temp)

- Preheat the oven to 180°C/Fan 160°C /350°F/Gas mark 4. Line a baking tray with baking parchment or a silicone sheet.

- Place the ground almonds, psyllium husks, baking powder and salt in a large bowl. Stir together thoroughly so that the psyllium is evenly distributed.

- Pour in the boiling water; it will froth up. Then immediately stir through and allow to rest for 5 minutes.

- Put 1 teaspoon of the cider vinegar in a clean glass bowl. Add the 2 egg whites and whisk until they form soft peaks. Incorporate the second teaspoon of cider vinegar. Fold the egg whites into the psyllium mixture. Don't worry if this is a gloopy mess at this stage – it's supposed to be like that!

- Use a dessertspoon to place 1 scoop of mix on the baking tray. Smooth with the back of the spoon to make a disc the size of a saucer. Have a cup of just boiled water standing by to dunk the spoon in to stop the dough sticking. Repeat until you have 6 discs on your tray.

- Bake in the oven for 45 minutes. Then turn it off and leave in the oven for at least another 15 minutes. Transfer to a wire rack to cool.

- For added convenience, you can freeze these flatbreads when cool and toast from frozen.

SWEET 'N' SALTY POPCORN

Wheat & Gluten Free ✓	Lactose Free ✓	Nightshade Free ✓
Gassy Veg Free ✓	Red Meat Free ✓	

Serves 4 / Ready in 25 minutes

100g (3½oz) popped corn

1 tbsp mild (light) olive oil

½ tsp salt

1 tbsp caster (fine) sugar

- Preheat the oven to 150°C/Fan 130°C/300°F/Gas mark 2.

- Place the popped corn in a large bowl and pour the olive oil over. Stir well until you have a very light coating of oil on all the corn.

- Tip the popped corn onto a baking tray and distribute evenly.

- On one half of the tray, sprinkle over the salt; do a little at a time making sure none of the corn gets too much.

- On the other half of the tray, sprinkle over the sugar. Again, try and distribute it evenly over the corn.

- Bake in the oven for 20 minutes – do not stir.

- Cool completely on the baking tray. When the popcorn is completely cool, gently mix the flavours together and place in an airtight jar. The popcorn keeps for up to 5 days.

PARMESAN POPCORN

Wheat & Gluten Free ✓	Lactose Free ✓	Nightshade Free ✓
Gassy Veg Free ✓	Red Meat Free ✓	

Serves 4 / Ready in 20 minutes

2 tsp olive oil

1 tsp garlic oil

½ tsp salt

½ tsp dried mixed herbs

30g (1oz) Parmesan, finely grated

100g popped corn

- Preheat the oven to 150°C/Fan 130°C/300°F/Gas mark 2.
- Mix together the olive oil, garlic oil, salt, mixed herbs and Parmesan.
- Place the popped corn in a large bowl and add the seasoned oil. Stir or toss gently to combine.
- Spread on 1 or 2 large baking trays. Bake for 15 minutes.
- Serve warm or cool and store in an airtight container for up to two days.

FRUITY FLAPJACKS

Wheat & Gluten Free ✓	Lactose Free ✓	Nightshade Free ✓
Gassy Veg Free ✓	Red Meat Free ✓	

Makes 16 / Ready in 40 minutes

1 orange, zest and juice

zest of 1 lemon

juice of ½ lemon

50g (2oz) golden syrup

200g (7oz) butter, plus extra for greasing

75g (3oz) soft brown sugar

1 ripe banana, peeled and mashed

250g (9oz) jumbo oats

100g (3½ oz) buckwheat flour

100g (3½ oz) pumpkin seeds

- Preheat the oven to 170°C/Fan 150°C/325°F/Gas mark 3. Line the bottom of a large baking tin with greaseproof (waxed) paper. Grease with a little butter.

- Place the orange and lemon zests in a saucepan. Add the golden syrup, butter and soft brown sugar. Heat gently until the butter has melted and the sugar has dissolved.

- Remove from the heat and stir in the orange and lemon juice plus the mashed banana.

- Mix together the oats, flour and pumpkin seeds in a large bowl.

- Pour the melted butter mixture into the oats. Mix together thoroughly.

- Spread the mixture out in the lined tin. Press down firmly with the back of a spoon.

- Bake for 25–30 minutes until just browned on top. Remove from the oven and cool for 5 minutes before cutting into squares, then leave to set and cool completely.

MINI COCONUT CAKES

Wheat & Gluten Free ✓	Lactose Free ✓	Nightshade Free ✓
Gassy Veg Free ✓	Red Meat Free ✓	

Makes 8–12 cakes / Ready in 20 minutes

60g (2oz) desiccated (dry unsweetened) coconut
60g (2oz) ground almonds
1 tbsp maple syrup
1 tbsp coconut oil
1 egg white
25g (1oz) dark chocolate, chopped

- Preheat the oven to 190°C/Fan 170°C/375°F/Gas mark 5. Line a baking tray with baking parchment.

- Place the coconut and ground almonds in a large bowl and stir well.

- In a small pan, heat the maple syrup and coconut oil together until the syrup has melted into the oil. Stir into the coconut and almonds.

- In a separate bowl, use an electric whisk to beat the egg white until it forms stiff peaks. Stir about a third of the egg white into the coconut mixture and then gently fold in the rest.

- Take heaped dessertspoonfuls (or an ice-cream scoop) of the mixture and place on the baking tray. This mixture makes 8–12 little cakes.

- Press a little dark chocolate into the middle of each cake and bake in the oven for 12–15 minutes until the edges are browned. Remove and transfer to a cooling rack.

INTRODUCING …
MILK

Note: In all of the 'Introducing …' chapters, ingredients in bold indicate trigger foods.

BUCKWHEAT PANCAKES WITH CRUSHED AVOCADO AND POACHED EGG

Wheat & Gluten Free ✓	Lactose Free ✗	Nightshade Free ✓
Gassy Veg Free ✓	Red Meat Free ✓	

Serves 2 / Ready in 15 minutes

For the pancakes:

1 large egg

90g buckwheat flour

1 tsp baking powder

½ tsp salt

300ml (½ pint) **milk**

1 tbsp mild (light) olive oil

For the topping:

2 eggs

1 ripe avocado, peeled and stoned (pitted)

juice of ½ lemon

salt and freshly ground black pepper

- In a large bowl or jug, whisk 1 egg until frothy. Add buckwheat flour, baking powder, salt and milk. Beat well to make a smooth batter. Leave to rest for a few minutes while you start the poached eggs for the topping.

- Half fill a wide saucepan with water about 2.5cm/1in deep. Heat the water until it is bubbling gently from the base of the pan, then carefully crack 1 egg on the side of the pan and lower gently into the water. Repeat with the other egg. Check that the water is still bubbling, but only just, then set a timer for 1 minute. At the end of the minute, turn off the heat and leave the eggs in the hot water for another 10 minutes. For an even simpler microwave-poached egg, check out the recipe in Step Up section (see page 147).

- Heat half the oil in a heavy-based frying pan (skillet) on a medium heat and wait for the oil to be hot but not smoky. Pour in half the batter and roll gently round the pan until it is a circle about the size of a saucer. Leave undisturbed for a minute or two, before turning when the underside is golden. Cook the other side. Transfer to a warm plate and repeat with the remaining batter.

- Place the avocado on a plate and mash lightly with a fork. Stir in the lemon juice.
- When you are ready to serve the dish, place the pancakes on 2 separate plates. Distribute the avocado between the 2 pancakes, season with salt and pepper and place the poached eggs on top.

BLUEBERRY OAT MUFFINS

Wheat & Gluten Free ✓	Lactose Free ✗	Nightshade Free ✓
Gassy Veg Free ✓	Red Meat Free ✓	

Makes 6 / Ready in 40 minutes

1 tsp mild (light) olive oil
1 ripe banana
1 egg
½ tsp vanilla essence
2 tbsp honey
1 tsp cinnamon
a pinch of salt
100g (3½oz) **Greek yogurt**
250ml (9fl oz) **milk**
140g (5oz) rolled oats (oatmeal)
100g (3½oz) blueberries

- Preheat the oven to 190°C/Fan 170°C /375°F/Gas mark 5. Dip kitchen paper (paper towels) into the mild (light) olive oil and wipe round each hole of a 6-hole muffin tin.
- In a medium-sized bowl, mash the banana until smooth. Beat in the egg.
- Add the vanilla essence, honey, cinnamon, salt and Greek yogurt. Mix together thoroughly, then stir in the milk and oats.
- Place a generous tablespoon of the batter into the base of each tin. Add a few blueberries to each and then fill with the rest of the batter. If you have any remaining blueberries you can add them to the top.
- Bake in the oven for 30 minutes. Allow to cool for a few minutes and eat warm.

HOT SMOKED SALMON WITH COLESLAW

Wheat & Gluten Free ✓	Lactose Free ✗	Nightshade Free ✓
Gassy Veg Free ✓	Red Meat Free ✓	

Serves 2 / Ready in 25 minutes

2 x 125g (4oz) lightly smoked salmon fillets

1 tsp olive oil

2 tbsp **Greek yogurt**

1 tbsp **milk**

1 tbsp good-quality mayonnaise

a pinch of salt

3 medium carrots (200g/7oz), finely grated or spiralized

1 bulb fennel, finely grated or spiralized

1 small apple, cored and thinly sliced

salt and freshly ground black pepper

- Preheat the oven to 180°C/Fan 160°C/350°F/Gas mark 4.

- Place the salmon fillets on a baking tray, season with salt and pepper and drizzle with olive oil. Bake in the oven for 15–20 minutes until cooked.

- Mix together the yogurt, milk, mayonnaise and salt and set aside. Combine the carrot, fennel and apple. Reserve 2 teaspoons of the yogurt dressing, then pour the remainder over the coleslaw and mix lightly.

- Distribute the coleslaw between 2 serving plates, place the baked salmon on the top and top each with a teaspoon of the dressing.

HALLOUMI AND ORANGE SALAD

Wheat & Gluten Free ✓	Lactose Free ✗	Nightshade Free ✓
Gassy Veg Free ✓	Red Meat Free ✓	

Serves 2 / Ready in 5 minutes

1 tbsp extra-virgin olive oil

250g (9oz) **halloumi,** drained and dried on kitchen paper

1 medium orange, peeled and divided into segments

juice of ½ orange

2 tsp apple cider vinegar

80g (3oz) watercress salad

salt and freshly ground black pepper

- Take a large griddle or frying (skillet) pan. Wipe round with a little of the olive oil on kitchen paper and heat to a high heat.

- Slice the halloumi into 8 pieces and griddle or fry for a couple of minutes on each side until lightly charred.

- In small bowl, combine the orange segments, orange juice, cider vinegar, remaining olive oil and salt and pepper.

- Arrange the watercress salad over 2 plates and divide the orange segments between them. Top with the griddled halloumi then pour over the rest of the dressing.

INTRODUCING ...
RED MEAT

SWEET CITRUS PORK

Wheat & Gluten Free ✓	Lactose Free ✓	Nightshade Free ✓
Gassy Veg Free ✓	Red Meat Free ✗	

Serves 2 / Ready in 25 minutes

2 tsp olive oil

2 × 125g (4oz) lean **pork steaks**

½ tsp asafoetida

1 tbsp cranberry jelly

zest and juice of 1 orange

1 tsp apple cider vinegar

1 heaped tsp butter

salt and freshly ground black pepper

- Heat the oil in a large frying pan (skillet) over a medium heat. Add the pork steaks and season generously with salt and pepper. Fry for 2 minutes on each side. At this stage, the pork should be browned but not cooked through.

- Add the asafoetida, cranberry jelly, orange zest and juice and the vinegar. Bring to a gentle simmer and stir to dissolve the cranberry jelly. Simmer for 5 minutes, turning the pork halfway through, until the meat is cooked.

- Remove the pork from the pan with a slotted spoon. Turn the heat up to medium and stir in the butter. Bubble for 2 minutes until the sauce is glossy.

- Arrange pork in a serving dish and pour the sauce over.

SUCCULENT STEAK WITH TANGY LEMON QUINOA

Wheat & Gluten Free ✓	Lactose Free ✓	Nightshade Free ✓
Gassy Veg Free ✓	Red Meat Free ✗	

Serves 2 / Ready in 30 minutes

1 tsp garlic oil

2 spring onions (scallions), green parts only, finely chopped

1 carrot, peeled and finely diced

100g (3½oz) (dried weight) quinoa

½ tsp asafoetida

½ tsp white pepper

zest and juice of 1 lemon

a pinch of salt

250ml (9fl oz) boiling water

2 × 100g (3½oz) **beef fillet or rump steaks**

1 tsp balsamic vinegar

50g (1¾oz) rocket (arugula)

salt and freshly ground black pepper

- Heat the garlic oil in a medium, lidded saucepan over a medium heat. Add the green part of the spring onions (scallions) and diced carrot. Stir-fry for 2 minutes. Stir in the quinoa, asafoetida, white pepper, lemon zest and a pinch of salt.

- Add the hot water to the quinoa and stir once. Put the lid on the pan, turn the heat down as low as possible and cook very gently for about 15 minutes. When cooked all the liquid will have been absorbed and the quinoa will be tender with just a little bite.

- While the quinoa is cooking, heat the grill (broiler) to a high setting.

- Season the steaks with salt and pepper and place under the hot grill. The cooking time will depend on thickness and desired degree of doneness. Anything from 5–10 minutes on each side.

- Set the steaks aside and cover for 5 minutes; resting makes the meat more tender.

- When both the steak and quinoa are done, stir the balsamic vinegar and half the lemon juice into the quinoa, then stir in the rocket (arugula).

- Serve with the steak resting on top of the quinoa and a little of the remaining lemon juice.

MINTED LAMB WITH BUTTERNUT CRUSH

Wheat & Gluten Free ✓	Lactose Free ✓	Nightshade Free ✓
Gassy Veg Free ✓	Red Meat Free ✗	

Serves 2 / Ready in 30 minutes

300g (11oz) (cut weight) butternut squash, cubed

1 tsp olive oil

2 fresh mint leaves

1 large bunch of flat-leaf (Italian) parsley

juice of 1 lemon

1 tsp garlic oil

1 tbsp extra-virgin olive oil

2 × 90g (3¼oz) lean **lamb leg steaks**

salt and freshly ground black pepper

- Preheat the oven to 220°C/Fan 200°C/425°F/Gas mark 7.

- Arrange the butternut squash on a baking tray and drizzle the teaspoon of olive oil over the top. Bake in the oven for 20 minutes.

- Meanwhile, place a little salt, the mint, parsley and lemon juice in a blender and process until they form a paste. If you don't have a blender, you can chop the ingredients finely instead. Gradually pour in the garlic oil and extra-virgin olive oil, blending until it forms a smooth emulsified sauce. Transfer the sauce to a wide dish that is big enough to hold the lamb.

- Preheat the grill (broiler) to medium–high. Season the lamb and place under the grill. Cook for 5–8 minutes on each side, depending on how you like your lamb. It should be seared on the outside and if you like it a little pink, you should make sure the inside gets properly hot – 145°C/293°F on a meat thermometer.

- Transfer the lamb to the serving dish and scoop up the sauce over the top. Leave to rest in the sauce for a few minutes before serving.

- Remove the butternut from the oven and use the back of a fork to lightly crush it. Divide between 2 plates and arrange the lamb over the top.

MAPLE BAKED PORK

Wheat & Gluten Free ✓	Lactose Free ✓	Nightshade Free ✓
Gassy Veg Free ✓	Red Meat Free ✗	

Serves 2 / Ready in 1 hour

2 × 125g (4oz) **pork** chops or steaks

1 tsp garlic oil

juice of ½ lemon

½ tsp asafoetida

1 tbsp maple syrup

100ml (3½fl oz) red wine

1 tbsp tamari sauce

1 tbsp apple cider vinegar

1 tsp cornflour (cornstarch), blended with a little water

½ tsp ground ginger

1 tsp English mustard

salt and freshly ground black pepper

- Preheat the oven to 200°C/Fan 180°C/400°F/Gas mark 6.

- Place the pork chops in a small roasting tin. Drizzle over the garlic oil and lemon juice. Season well with the asafoetida and salt and pepper.

- Bake for 20 minutes.

- Meanwhile, mix together the maple syrup, red wine, tamari sauce, cider vinegar, blended cornflour (cornstarch), ground ginger and English mustard.

- Remove the pork from the oven and pour the sauce over, giving everything a good coating.

- Bake for a further 30 minutes, basting every 10 minutes.

- Serve the pork with the sauce spooned over.

SPRING CHICKEN STEW

Wheat & Gluten Free ✓	Lactose Free ✓	Nightshade Free ✓
Gassy Veg Free ✓	Red Meat Free ✗	

Serves 2 / Ready in 45 minutes

50g (2oz) chopped **streaky bacon** or **lardons**

2 skinless, boneless chicken thighs, about 360g (12oz)

1 carrot, peeled and chopped

2 celery sticks, finely sliced

1 tsp mixed dried herbs

200ml (7fl oz) dry (hard) cider

250ml (9fl oz) water

80g (3oz) frozen peas

1 tbsp Dijon mustard

1 Little Gem (Boston) lettuce, roughly shredded

1 small handful of fresh tarragon (optional)

salt and freshly ground black pepper

- Heat the chopped bacon or lardons in a heavy-based lidded saucepan, cooking them until they are brown all over. Remove the meat from the pan with a slotted spoon and set aside. Add the chicken thighs and cook on the first side for about 5 minutes over a medium heat.

- Turn the chicken over and add the carrot, celery and dried herbs. Give everything a stir and continue to cook for a further 5 minutes. Return the chopped bacon or lardons to the pan.

- Pour in the cider and water. Then add the peas. Bring to the boil, then reduce the heat, put the lid on and cook for 20–30 minutes until the chicken is cooked through.

- Remove the lid, stir in the mustard and season with salt and pepper. Finally, toss the lettuce and tarragon, if using, over the chicken and let them wilt into the sauce for about 2 minutes.

- Serve immediately.

COTTAGE PIE

Wheat & Gluten Free ✓	Lactose Free ✓	Nightshade Free ✓
Gassy Veg Free ✓	Red Meat Free ✗	

Serves 6 / Ready in about 2 hours

1 tbsp olive oil

3 carrots, peeled and diced

2 parsnips, peeled and diced

4 celery sticks, trimmed and diced

1kg (2lb 3oz) lean **minced beef**

2 bay leaves

500ml (18fl oz) water

1 heaped tsp cornflour (cornstarch), blended with a little water

1 heaped tsp Dijon mustard

1 tsp Worcestershire sauce

1 tbsp tamari sauce

500g (1lb 2oz) sweet potato, 3–4 depending on size, cut into chunks

1 tbsp butter

30g (1oz) mature Cheddar cheese, grated

salt and freshly ground black pepper

- Heat the olive oil in a large, wide casserole dish. Add the carrots, parsnips and celery and fry lightly in the oil for 2 minutes. Crumble in the minced beef. Keep stirring the beef and squashing any lumps until none of the meat is pink.

- Add the bay leaves and water and bring up to a simmer. When simmering, slowly stir in the cornflour (cornstarch). Then season well with salt and pepper. Add the mustard, Worcestershire sauce and tamari sauce. Put the lid on the pan and cook on the lowest heat for about an hour. Alternatively, transfer to a low oven (160°C/Fan 140°C/325°F/Gas mark 3) for an hour.

- Meanwhile, boil the sweet potato in water for about 15 minutes until tender. Drain and mash with the butter.

- Turn up the oven to 200°C/Fan 180°C/400°F/Gas mark 6.

- Scoop the sweet potato on top of the minced beef and smooth with the back of a fork. Sprinkle over the Cheddar and bake in the oven for 35–40 minutes.

INTRODUCING ...
NIGHTSHADE

CHICKEN CAESAR SALAD

Wheat & Gluten Free ✓	Lactose Free ✓	Nightshade Free ✗
Gassy Veg Free ✓	Red Meat Free ✓	

Serves 1 / Ready in 15 minutes

1 x 125g (4oz) skinless chicken breast fillet, cubed

1 tsp olive oil

1 cos (romaine) lettuce, washed and outer leaves removed

4 **cherry tomatoes**, halved

1 tbsp good-quality mayonnaise

1 tsp extra-virgin olive oil

10g (1 heaped tbsp) Parmesan cheese, finely grated

1 tsp apple cider vinegar

1 tsp capers

4 large black olives

freshly ground black pepper

- In a small frying pan (skillet), fry the chicken in the olive oil until the chicken is cooked through, so that the juices run clear when cut.

- Chop the lettuce into ribbons about 1cm (½in) wide and place in a wide bowl. Add the cherry tomatoes.

- In a small bowl, mix together the mayonnaise, extra-virgin olive oil, half the Parmesan, vinegar and capers.

- Stir the mayonnaise mixture gently into the lettuce and transfer to a serving bowl.

- Add the chicken and toss through.

- Finally, add the black olives and sprinkle with the remaining Parmesan cheese and a dash of black pepper.

CORIANDER CHICKEN CURRY

Wheat & Gluten Free ✓	Lactose Free ✓	Nightshade Free ✗
Gassy Veg Free ✓	Red Meat Free ✓	

Serves 2 / Ready in 15 minutes

1 tbsp garlic oil

1 large thumb (5cm/2in) fresh ginger, peeled, finely grated and mixed with 1 tbsp water

1 **red chilli**, deseeded if preferred and finely chopped

¼ tsp **cayenne pepper**

½ tsp ground cumin

½ tsp ground coriander

½ tsp turmeric

½ tsp salt

2 skinless chicken breast fillets (about 125g/4oz each), cubed

1 large bunch of fresh coriander (cilantro), chopped

juice of 1 lemon, freshly squeezed

300ml (½ pint) water

- Heat the garlic oil on a low–medium heat in a lidded saucepan. Add the ginger and, stirring continuously, heat for 1–2 minutes. Add the chilli, cayenne, cumin, ground coriander, turmeric and salt. Stir well for a further minute.

- Add the chicken to the pan and mix well, making sure the chicken pieces are well coated. Add most of the chopped coriander (cilantro), reserving a little; add the lemon juice and water. Bring to the boil, put the lid on the pan and reduce the heat to minimum. Cook on a low heat for 12 minutes, turning the chicken halfway through, until the meat is cooked through and tender, so that the juices run clear when cut.

- Serve with the remaining coriander (cilantro) sprinkled on top.

SWEET ITALIAN TURKEY SAUSAGE

Wheat & Gluten Free ✓	Lactose Free ✓	Nightshade Free ✗
Gassy Veg Free ✓	Red Meat Free ✓	

Serves 4 (Makes 12 meatballs or 4 sausages) / Ready in 5 minutes
(plus 10/30 minutes chilling)

500g (1lb 2oz) turkey thigh mince

1 tbsp olive oil

1 tsp salt

1 tsp pepper

1 tsp oregano

1 tsp dried mixed herbs

1 tsp asafoetida

1 tsp **paprika**

1 tsp **mild chilli powder**

1 tbsp **ketchup**

- Place the turkey in a large bowl. Add the salt, pepper, herbs, asafoetida, paprika, chilli powder and ketchup.

- Use your hands to pound and mix the ingredients together. Make sure the mince is thoroughly broken up.

- Form the meat into 4 sausages or 12 meatballs. Place on a tray in the freezer for 10 minutes or in the fridge for 30 minutes before cooking.

- To cook, lightly fry in a tablespoon olive oil. If you're adding to a sauce (for example, page 192), you can fry the meatballs for about 4 minutes and then add the sauce and leave to bubble for about 10 minutes. Burgers or sausages take about 10 minutes, turning once.

ALL-IN-ONE SUMMER MEATBALL STEW

Wheat & Gluten Free ✓	Lactose Free ✓	Nightshade Free ✗
Gassy Veg Free ✓	Red Meat Free ✓	

Serves 4 / Ready in 30 minutes

1 tbsp garlic oil

12 Sweet Italian Turkey Sausage meatballs (see page 191)

1 carrot, peeled and chopped

2 celery sticks, finely sliced

2 parsnips, peeled and diced

500g new potatoes, halved

1 tsp mixed dried herbs

1 bay leaf

1 tbsp **tomato purée**

1 tbsp **ketchup**

1 tsp English mustard

1 tsp salt

1 litre (1¾fl oz) No-fuss 'Safe' Stock (see page 142)

1 litre (1¾fl oz) water

2 **tomatoes**, roughly chopped

- Heat the garlic oil on a medium heat in a wide, shallow saucepan. Add the meatballs and fry for 4–5 minutes, turning once, until browned all over. Remove from the pan with a slotted spoon and set aside.

- Add the carrot, celery, parsnips and new potatoes to the pan and stir through. Put the dried herbs, bay leaf, tomato purée, ketchup, mustard and salt on the top. Pour in the stock and water and bring up to the boil. Simmer for 10 minutes.

- Drop the meatballs into the stew, one by one, and cook for a further 15–20 minutes.

- Remove from the heat and take out the bay leaf. Use a slotted spoon to pull out 4 or 5 potatoes and a few carrots. Crush them with the back of a fork and return them to the pan; add the tomatoes. Cover and allow the sauce to rest and thicken for a few minutes before serving.

FAST CHICKEN SALAD

Wheat & Gluten Free ✓	Lactose Free ✓	Nightshade Free ✗
Gassy Veg Free ✓	Red Meat Free ✓	

Serves 1 / Ready in 10 minutes

1 × 150g (5oz) skinless chicken breast fillet, cut into 4–5 slices

1 heaped tsp cornflour (cornstarch)

salt and freshly ground black pepper

¾ tsp **paprika**

1 tsp olive oil

1 × 100g (3½oz) bag baby leaf salad

100g (3½oz) cucumber (about 5cm/2in), roughly chopped

10 **cherry tomatoes**, halved

For the dressing:

2 tsp mayonnaise

1 tsp extra-virgin olive oil

a pinch of salt

- Place the chicken in a bowl and sprinkle on the cornflour (cornstarch), salt and pepper and ½ teaspoon paprika. Use your hands to toss the chicken in the flour and make sure it is evenly covered.

- Heat the oil in a frying pan (skillet) over a medium heat. When hot, add the chicken and fry for about 4 minutes on each side, depending on thickness.

- Meanwhile, prepare all your salad ingredients and place in a serving bowl. Combine the mayonnaise, extra-virgin olive oil, pinch of salt and remaining ¼ teaspoon paprika in a small cup.

- Place the just cooked chicken on top of the salad and drizzle the dressing over.

CHILLI BAKED SALMON

Wheat & Gluten Free ✓	Lactose Free ✓	Nightshade Free ✗
Gassy Veg Free ✓	Red Meat Free ✓	

Serves 2 / Ready in 20 minutes

2 skinless, boneless salmon fillets

1 heaped tsp cornflour (cornstarch)

1 tbsp water

1 tsp brown sugar

1 tsp **chilli flakes**

¼ tsp ground ginger

1 tsp red wine vinegar

zest and juice of 1 lime

salt and freshly ground black pepper

- Preheat the oven to 200°C/180°C/400°F/Gas mark 6.

- Put a large piece of foil on a baking tray. Put the salmon fillets on the foil at least 2.5cm (1 inch) apart. Pull up the sides of the foil to make a loose parcel around the salmon.

- Bake for 15 minutes.

- Meanwhile, place the cornflour (cornstarch) in a small bowl or cup. Add the water a little at a time to make a smooth paste. Add the brown sugar, chilli flakes, ginger, red wine vinegar and lime zest and juice.

- Remove the salmon from the oven and peel back the foil. Rub the chilli glaze all over the top and sides of the salmon. Leaving the foil open, bake in the oven for a further 5 minutes.

SIMPLEST PASTA BAKE

Wheat & Gluten Free ✓	Lactose Free ✓	Nightshade Free ✗
Gassy Veg Free ✓	Red Meat Free ✓	

Serves 4 / Ready in 30 minutes

500g (1lb 2oz) buckwheat pasta

500ml (18fl oz) water

2 x 400g (14oz) tins **chopped tomatoes**

2 tbsp garlic oil

½ tsp asafoetida

1 tsp salt

2 x 160g (5oz) tins tuna, drained

120g (4oz) mature Cheddar cheese, grated

freshly ground black pepper

- Preheat the oven to 190°C/Fan 170°C/375°F/Gas mark 5.

- Place the pasta, water, chopped tomatoes, garlic oil, asafoetida and salt in a large saucepan. Bring to the boil, stir once and simmer vigorously for 10 minutes.

- Stir once again and transfer half of the pasta to a wide baking dish. Layer on half the tuna and a little bit of cheese. Add the rest of the pasta, then the remaining tuna and finally finish with the remaining cheese. Season generously with the pepper.

- Bake in the oven for 15–20 minutes until the cheese bubbles on the top.

CHINESE PRAWN NOODLES

Wheat & Gluten Free ✓	Lactose Free ✓	Nightshade Free ✗
Gassy Veg Free ✓	Red Meat Free ✓	

Serves 2 / Ready in 20 minutes

1 tsp garlic oil

1 tsp Chinese five-spice powder

1 thumb ginger, peeled and finely grated

250g (9oz) raw king prawns (king or jumbo shrimp)

1 heaped tsp brown sugar

1 **red chilli**, deseeded and finely sliced

1 tsp **tomato purée** (paste)

4 spring onions (scallions), green parts only, sliced

200g (7oz) cooked rice noodles

juice of ½ lime

1 tsp fish sauce

1 tsp tamari sauce

1 small handful of fresh coriander (cilantro), chopped

- In a wok or large frying pan (skillet), heat the garlic oil on a medium heat. Add the five-spice powder, ginger, prawns (shrimp), brown sugar, red chilli, tomato purée and green parts of the spring onions (scallions). Stir-fry for 3–4 minutes until the prawns are pink.

- Add the rice noodles, lime juice, fish sauce, tamari sauce and fresh coriander (cilantro). Stir-fry for another 2 minutes until everything is piping hot. Serve immediately.

MEXICAN CHICKEN SOUP

Wheat & Gluten Free ✓	Lactose Free ✓	Nightshade Free ✗
Gassy Veg Free ✓	Red Meat Free ✓	

Serves 2 / Ready in 1 hour

2 chicken drumsticks
1 small carrot, peeled and roughly chopped
2 celery sticks, trimmed and finely chopped
500ml (18fl oz) water
1 x 400g (14oz) tin **chopped tomatoes**
1 **green (bell) pepper**, deseeded and chopped
1 tsp dried mixed herbs
½ tsp **paprika**
½ tsp **smoked paprika**
¼ tsp turmeric
¼ tsp ground cumin
½ tsp asafoetida
1 tsp salt
freshly ground black pepper
1 tsp **mild chilli powder**
1 large handful of flat-leaf parsley, stalks removed and chopped

- Place the chicken drumsticks, carrot and celery in a large saucepan. Pour over the water and bring to a simmer. Cook for 20 minutes, then remove the chicken drumsticks with a slotted spoon and set aside to cool.

- Add the chopped tomatoes, green (bell) pepper and bring back up to simmering point. Add the dried herbs, paprika, smoked paprika, turmeric, cumin, asafoetida, salt, black pepper and chilli powder, then simmer gently for 30 minutes.

- Remove the skin from the drumsticks and pull as much chicken as possible off the bone. Shred the chicken meat and return it to the soup in the pan. Remove from the heat, stir in the parsley and serve.

MUSHROOM-STUFFED PEPPERS

Wheat & Gluten Free ✓	Lactose Free ✓	Nightshade Free ✗
Gassy Veg Free ✓	Red Meat Free ✓	

Serves 1 / Ready in 15 minutes

1 **yellow (bell) pepper**

150g (5oz) mushrooms, washed

1 tsp olive oil

2 **sun-dried tomato** pieces in oil, chopped

½ tsp dried Italian herbs

30g (1oz) feta cheese, crumbled

salt and freshly ground black pepper

- Preheat the oven to 220°C/Fan 200°C/425°F/Gas mark 7.

- Wash the pepper and halve lengthways, leaving the stalk attached. Cut away the inside of the stalk together with all the seeds. Place the 2 halves open-side down on a baking tray and cook for 10 minutes.

- Meanwhile, pull the stalks off the mushrooms and finely chop them. Slice the mushrooms.

- Heat the oil in a wide frying pan (skillet) and add the mushrooms (stalks and slices). Fry for 2–4 minutes until soft and glossy. Remove from the heat. Stir the sun-dried tomatoes, dried herbs and salt and pepper into the mushrooms.

- Remove the peppers from the oven and carefully turn them over with a fish slice. Scoop up the mushroom mixture and push it gently into the peppers. Sprinkle the feta over the top. Return to the oven for another 5 minutes. Serve immediately.

MEDITERRANEAN CHICKEN

Wheat & Gluten Free ✓	Lactose Free ✓	Nightshade Free ✗
Gassy Veg Free ✓	Red Meat Free ✓	

Serves 2 / Ready in 25 minutes

2 × 150g (5oz) skinless, boneless chicken breast fillets

1 tbsp **tomato purée** (paste)

1 small handful of fresh basil, torn

1 tsp garlic oil

1 × 400g (14oz) tin **whole tomatoes**

a pinch of salt

1 tbsp red wine vinegar

25g (1oz) feta cheese, lightly crumbled

8–10 large black olives, pitted and halved

- Cut each chicken breast into 2 pieces and lightly score on both sides. Rub the tomato purée (paste) and half the basil over the 4 pieces of chicken and leave to rest while you prepare the sauce.

- Heat the garlic oil gently in a non-stick saucepan. Add the tinned tomatoes, salt and the remaining basil and simmer over a medium heat for 10 minutes. Reduce the heat and break up the tomatoes with the back of a wooden spoon. Add the red wine vinegar and continue to simmer gently for another 10 minutes.

- Meanwhile, preheat the grill (broiler) to medium. Arrange the chicken pieces on the grill pan and grill (broil) for 7–8 minutes on each side. The chicken should be cooked through so that the juices run clear when cut, and turning golden all over.

- Add the chicken, half the feta and half the olives to the tomato sauce and stir in. Heat for a further 2–3 minutes. Serve with the rest of the feta and olives sprinkled over the top.

CHERRY TOMATO PASTA

Wheat & Gluten Free ✓	Lactose Free ✓	Nightshade Free ✗
Gassy Veg Free ✓	Red Meat Free ✓	

Serves 4 / Ready in 20 minutes

200g (7oz) buckwheat pasta

200g (7oz) new potatoes, quartered

1 tsp white pepper

1 tsp salt

1 tsp asafoetida

½ tsp **chilli flakes**

1 bay leaf

1 tbsp **tomato purée (paste)**

1 tsp dried mixed Italian herbs

1 litre (1¾ pints) water

1 tbsp garlic oil

200g (7oz) green beans, trimmed

200g (7oz) **cherry tomatoes**, halved

1 heaped tsp cornflour (cornstarch), blended with a little water

lashings of Parmesan and black pepper, to serve

- Take a wide and lidded shallow pan. Add the pasta and new potatoes. Put the white pepper, salt, asafoetida, chilli flakes, bay leaf, tomato purée and dried mixed herbs on top. Pour in the water. Bring to the boil, then reduce the heat and simmer for 10 minutes until the pasta and potatoes are nearly tender.

- Stir through the garlic oil, green beans and cherry tomatoes. Put the lid on the pan and continue to cook on the lowest heat for 5 minutes.

- Add the blended cornflour (cornstarch) and stir through thoroughly. Put the lid back on and leave to stand for a few minutes to thicken.

- Serve with a generous serving of Parmesan and black pepper.

ROASTED AUBERGINE PASTA

Wheat & Gluten Free ✓	Lactose Free ✓	Nightshade Free ✗
Gassy Veg Free ✓	Red Meat Free ✓	

Serves 2 / Ready in 15 minutes

1 large **aubergine** (eggplant), cut into chunks

2 tbsp garlic oil

200g (7oz) buckwheat pasta

300g (11oz) **cherry tomatoes**, halved

1 tbsp balsamic vinegar

1 tsp granulated sugar

1 handful of fresh basil leaves, torn

salt and freshly ground black pepper

- Preheat the oven to 220°C/Fan 200°C/425°F/Gas mark 7. Tip the aubergine (eggplant) into a roasting tin. Pour in the garlic oil and toss through with your hands. Season generously with salt and pepper. Roast for 10 minutes.

- Meanwhile, cook the pasta according to the packet instructions, then drain.

- Add the cherry tomatoes, balsamic vinegar and sugar to the roasting tin. Bake for another 5 minutes. Add the basil leaves to the tray, stir and squash a few of the tomatoes with the back of the spoon. Tip the pasta into the roasting tin and stir everything together. Divide between 2 bowls and serve.

ADVENTURE RECIPES: MILK, RED MEAT AND NIGHTSHADE

WARM SALAD OF ASPARAGUS AND BACON

Wheat & Gluten Free ✓	Lactose Free ✓	Nightshade Free ✗
Gassy Veg Free ✓	Red Meat Free ✗	

Serves 1 / Ready in 15 minutes

1 large egg, pricked at the big end with a pin

100g (3½oz) fine asparagus

1 slice smoked **bacon**

8 **cherry tomatoes**, halved

1 tsp extra-virgin olive oil

1 tsp balsamic vinegar

salt and freshly ground black pepper

- Bring a small saucepan of water to a fast boil. Slowly lower the egg into the water and cook for 7½ minutes. Remove the egg from the water and peel under cold running water. Set aside.

- Lightly cook the asparagus by plunging into boiling water for 4–5 minutes, until just tender.

- Fry the bacon for several minutes until cooked and crispy. Drain on kitchen paper.

- Mix together the cherry tomatoes with the olive oil and balsamic vinegar.

- Put the asparagus on a plate and pour the cherry tomatoes over.

- Quarter the egg and add it to the pile. Season with salt and pepper. Finally, add the bacon to the top of the pile.

QUICK ITALIAN BEEF STEW

Wheat & Gluten Free ✓	Lactose Free ✓	Nightshade Free ✗
Gassy Veg Free ✓	Red Meat Free ✗	

Serves 2 / Ready in 30 minutes

1 tsp garlic oil

200g (7oz) lean **beef strips**

2 spring onions (scallions), green parts only, chopped

1 **yellow (bell) pepper**, deseeded and sliced

1 × 400g (14oz) tin **chopped tomatoes**

½ tsp asafoetida

½ tsp dried mixed herbs

a little fresh oregano (optional)

12 large black olives, pitted

salt and freshly ground black pepper

- Heat the oil in a large pan over a high heat. Season the beef with salt and pepper. When the oil is hot, toss in the beef and stir-fry for 2 minutes. Remove the beef from the pan and set aside.

- Reduce the heat to medium and fry the green part of the spring onions (scallions) and the (bell) pepper for 5 minutes. With the heat still at medium, add the tomatoes, asafoetida and herbs and simmer for 15 minutes.

- Stir through the beef strips and olives and heat for a further 2 minutes before serving.

GREEK ROASTED AUBERGINE

Wheat & Gluten Free ✓	Lactose Free ✗	Nightshade Free ✗
Gassy Veg Free ✓	Red Meat Free ✓	

Serves 2 / Ready in 20 minutes

1 large (or 2 small, about 400g/14 oz) **aubergine (eggplant)**, cut into thin slices

1 tbsp olive oil

salt and freshly ground black pepper

For the dressing:

3 tbsp **Greek yogurt**

juice of ½ lemon

½ tsp **paprika**

1 tsp garlic oil

1 small handful of fresh mint, chopped

- Preheat the oven to 220°C/Fan 200°C/425°F/Gas mark 7.

- Spread the aubergine slices over 2 baking trays and drizzle with olive oil. Season generously with salt and pepper. Roast in the oven for 20 minutes, turning halfway through cooking.

- Meanwhile, make up the dressing by combining the yogurt, lemon juice, paprika and garlic oil in a small bowl.

- When you are ready to serve, arrange the aubergine slices on a plate, drizzle the dressing over and top with the mint.

PORK IN CIDER

Wheat & Gluten Free ✓	Lactose Free ✗	Nightshade Free ✓
Gassy Veg Free ✓	Red Meat Free ✗	

Serves 2 / Ready in 15 minutes

2 x 125g (4oz) lean **pork steaks**

2 tsp garlic oil

200ml (7fl oz) dry (hard) cider

1 tbsp wholegrain mustard

2 tbsp **crème fraîche**

salt and freshly ground black pepper

- Place the pork steaks on a chopping board and tenderise (bash) with a meat tenderizer or rolling pin. Continue until the pork is less than 1cm/½in thin. Rub in the garlic oil and a little salt and pepper to both sides.

- Heat a frying pan (skillet) on a high heat and quick fry the pork until cooked through; depending on thickness, this should take between 6 and 8 minutes, turning once.

- Remove the pork from the pan and set aside to rest.

- Add the cider to the pan, bring to the boil and simmer vigorously for 5 minutes. Turn the heat down to low, then add the wholegrain mustard and crème fraîche. Stir, then put the pork back in the pan and heat for 2 minutes before serving.

FRESH SPINACH CURRY WITH PANEER

Wheat & Gluten Free ✓	Lactose Free ✗	Nightshade Free ✗
Gassy Veg Free ✓	Red Meat Free ✓	

Serves 2 / Ready in 10 minutes

1 tsp garlic oil

200g (7oz) **paneer**, cut into cubes

2 spring onions (scallions), green parts only, chopped

1 small thumb fresh ginger, peeled and cut into matchsticks

1 **green chilli**, deseeded and finely sliced

12 **cherry tomatoes**, halved

¼ tsp ground coriander

¼ tsp ground cumin

½ tsp asafoetida

100g (3½oz) fresh young spinach leaves

salt and freshly ground black pepper

- Heat the garlic oil in a wide, lidded frying pan (skillet) over a medium heat. Season the paneer generously with salt and pepper and toss into the pan with the spring onions. Fry for a few minutes until golden, stirring often. Remove from the pan with a slotted spoon and set aside.

- Reduce the heat and add the ginger and chilli. Add the cherry tomatoes, put the lid on the pan, and cook for 3–4 minutes.

- Add the ground coriander, ground cumin, asafoetida and stir. Return the paneer to the pan and stir until coated. Add the spinach on top of the paneer but do not stir in. Put the lid on and allow the spinach to wilt for no more than 1 minute, then stir together before serving.

INTRODUCING ...
GASSY VEGETABLES

HONEYED CHICKEN AND BROCCOLI

Wheat & Gluten Free ✓	Lactose Free ✓	Nightshade Free ✓
Gassy Veg Free ✗	Red Meat Free ✓	

Serves 2 / Ready in 15 minutes

juice of ½ lemon

1 tsp balsamic vinegar

2 tsp extra-virgin olive oil

2 tsp runny honey

1 tsp olive oil

2 × 150g (5oz) skinless chicken breast fillets, cut in half

1 head **broccoli**, about 150g (trimmed weight), cut into florets

salt and freshly ground black pepper

- Begin by preparing your serving dish. It should be wide with a lip and able to hold the chicken and broccoli comfortably. Put the lemon juice, vinegar, extra-virgin olive oil, honey and salt and pepper in the dish and whisk together with a fork. Set aside.

- Heat the olive oil in a frying pan (skillet) over a medium–high heat. When hot, add the chicken pieces and fry for 8–10 minutes until golden and cooked through so that the juices run clear when cooked. As soon as it is cooked, transfer to the serving dish and toss in the dressing.

- Meanwhile, bring a pan of water to the boil and plunge in the broccoli. Cook for 6 minutes until tender. Drain and combine with the chicken and dressing.

- Leave the dish for 2 minutes before serving to allow the flavours to combine.

CHICKEN WITH GINGER AND LENTILS

Wheat & Gluten Free ✓	Lactose Free ✓	Nightshade Free ✓
Gassy Veg Free ✗	Red Meat Free ✓	

Serves 2 / Ready in 15 minutes

2 × 150g (5oz) skinless chicken fillets, cut into chunks

1 tsp olive oil

1 heaped tsp butter

1 large thumb fresh ginger, peeled and finely grated

1 **garlic** clove, finely chopped

1 carrot, peeled and coarsely grated

200g (7fl oz) ready-to-eat **puy lentils**

salt and freshly ground black pepper

- Season the chicken with salt and pepper.

- Heat the olive oil and butter together in a wide frying pan (skillet) over a medium–high heat. When hot, toss in the chicken and fry for 6–8 minutes, turning once, until just cooked.

- Stir in the ginger, garlic and carrot and fry for 2 minutes before turning the heat to low. Add the lentils and stir. Cook slowly for a further few minutes until the lentils have warmed through.

CHICKEN SATAY

Wheat & Gluten Free ✓	Lactose Free ✓	Nightshade Free ✓
Gassy Veg Free ✗	Red Meat Free ✓	

Serves 2 / Ready in 10 minutes, plus 1 hour marinating

1 **shallot**, peeled and diced

1 **garlic clove**, peeled and crushed

1 thumb ginger, peeled and finely grated

1 level tbsp peanut butter

1 tsp runny honey

2 tbsp tamari sauce

250g (9oz) skinless chicken breast fillets, cut into cubes, about 2.5cm (1in) square

- To make the marinade, mix the shallot, garlic, ginger, peanut butter, honey and tamari sauce together in a bowl. Add the chicken and toss until it is coated all over in the marinade. Leave to marinate in the refrigerator for at least 1 hour.

- Preheat the grill (broiler) to medium or light the barbecue. Thread the chicken cubes onto 2–4 skewers, leaving room between each piece to allow them to cook thoroughly. Grill (broil) for about 10 minutes, turning regularly, until cooked through, so that the juices run clear when cut. Serve immediately.

LEEK AND POTATO FRITTATA

Wheat & Gluten Free ✓	Lactose Free ✓	Nightshade Free ✓
Gassy Veg Free ✗	Red Meat Free ✓	

Serves 2 / Ready in 30 minutes

2 tsp olive oil

2 **leeks**, trimmed and chopped

200g (7oz) new potatoes, diced

3 large eggs

½ tsp English mustard

50g (2fl oz) pecorino cheese, grated

freshly ground black pepper

- In a lidded frying pan (skillet), heat 1 teaspoon oil over a medium–high heat. Toss in the leeks and potatoes and stir-fry for 2 minutes. Reduce the heat, add 4 tablespoons water and put the lid on. Sweat the leeks and potatoes for 10–15 minutes or until tender. Allow to cool.
- Put the eggs and mustard in a bowl and whisk thoroughly. Stir in the grated cheese and cooled vegetables.
- Preheat the grill (broiler) to a medium setting.
- Choose a frying pan (skillet) with a metal handle that can go under the grill. Wipe with kitchen paper (paper towels) dipped in the remaining oil. Heat over a medium–high heat and, when hot, add the vegetable and egg mixture. Roll the pan around so the egg covers the base of the pan evenly. Immediately turn the heat to the lowest setting and cook, uncovered, for about 10 minutes or until the base and sides are firm.
- Sprinkle over the black pepper and put the pan under the grill for another 5–10 minutes until the top is firm and golden.
- Invert onto a plate and serve immediately or allow to cool and serve in wedges.

SWEET AND SOUR CHICKEN

Wheat & Gluten Free ✓	Lactose Free ✓	Nightshade Free ✓
Gassy Veg Free ✗	Red Meat Free ✓	

Serves 2 / Ready in 15 minutes

2 × 150g (5oz) skinless chicken fillets, cut into chunks

1 heaped tsp cornflour (cornstarch), seasoned with salt and freshly ground black
    pepper

2 tsp olive oil

1 **red onion**, peeled and quartered

1 carrot, peeled and diced

1 **garlic clove**, peeled and finely chopped

150g (5oz) sweetcorn

1 level tsp granulated sugar

1 tbsp white wine vinegar

1 tsp fish sauce

a few drops of Worcestershire sauce

1 tbsp tamari sauce

1 tbsp dry sherry

- Toss the chicken in the seasoned cornflour (cornstarch) until lightly
  coated.

- Heat the olive oil in a wide saucepan or wok over a medium–high heat.
  Add the chicken, red onion and carrot and stir-fry until the chicken is
  browned all over, about 7–8 minutes. Remove the chicken from the pan
  with a slotted spoon, cover and keep warm.

- Return the pan to a medium heat, add the garlic and sweetcorn and stir-
  fry for 3–4 minutes.

- Return the chicken to the pan and stir in the sugar, vinegar, fish sauce,
  Worcestershire sauce, tamari sauce, 50ml (2fl oz) water and the sherry.
  Simmer for 3 more minutes before serving.

PUY LENTIL AND FETA SALAD

Wheat & Gluten Free ✓	Lactose Free ✓	Nightshade Free ✓
Gassy Veg Free ✗	Red Meat Free ✓	

Serves 2 / Ready in 10 minutes

1 tsp balsamic vinegar

1 tbsp apple cider vinegar

1 tsp walnut oil

1 tsp extra-virgin olive oil

1 tsp English mustard

4 basil leaves, torn

freshly ground black pepper

1 x 400g (14oz) tin ready-to-eat **puy lentils**, drained

1 tbsp capers, drained

30g (1oz) rocket leaves (arugula)

150g (5oz) cooked sweetcorn

60g (2oz) feta cheese, crumbled

30g (1oz) walnuts, roughly chopped

- Prepare the dressing by mixing together the balsamic vinegar, cider vinegar, walnut oil, extra-virgin olive oil, English mustard, basil leaves and black pepper.

- In a large bowl, combine the lentils with the capers, rocket (arugula) and sweetcorn. Stir about two-thirds of the dressing through the lentils. Sprinkle the feta over the top and add the walnuts. Finally, drizzle over the rest of the dressing.

INTRODUCING ...
WHEAT AND GLUTEN

NUT AND SEED MUESLI

Wheat & Gluten Free ✕	Lactose Free ✓	Nightshade Free ✓
Gassy Veg Free ✓	Red Meat Free ✓	

This recipe introduces gluten in the form of barley flakes. These are really delicious and healthy. If you wanted to test whether you had a gluten intolerance versus a wheat intolerance, this is a good recipe to try. Remember, wheat always contains gluten but a recipe can contain other forms of gluten (barley gluten, in this case) that may not trigger your sensitivities.

Makes 10 x 50g (1½ oz) portions / Ready in 2 minutes
170g (6oz) jumbo oats
120g (4oz) **barley flakes**
120g (4oz) chopped dates
30g Brazil nuts, halved
30g whole almonds
30g sunflower seeds

- Tip all the ingredients into a large bowl. Give it a good stir and transfer to an airtight container.

The Gentle Reintroduction of Wheat using Kamut Ancient Flour

Kamut or Khorasan is an ancient grain, often called the 'Wheat of the Pharaohs'. Kamut is simply the brand name for organic Khorasan flour. Khorasan flour is used in exactly the same way as standard wheat; however, many people find it easier to tolerate, and so it is often used by those who are wheat intolerant. After several weeks with no wheat whatsoever, introducing Kamut bread is a great way to see if you will be able to reintroduce wheat back into your diet.

The gluten in Khorasan is slightly different to that which we find in modern wheat. It is extremely gentle on the digestive system and is less likely than standard wheat to cause symptoms such as bloating. But if you believe you are gluten intolerant (as opposed to wheat intolerant) you should not introduce Kamut wheat at this time.

The flavour of Khorasan baking is fabulous. It has a rich, buttery flavour and excellent texture and crust. As a bonus, it contains approximately 40 per cent more protein than normal wheat and more dietary fibre than wholemeal bread.

As always, keep everything in moderation – stick to only one meal a day containing Khorasan wheat. If you love bread and want to reintroduce it into your diet, then try these amazing recipes. And the really, really good news is – this is real bread and tastes magnificent.

Here you'll find recipes for Kamut Daily Loaf, Kamut Quick Rolls, Kamut Flatbreads and Kamut Pizza Dough.

KAMUT DAILY LOAF

This recipe is for you if you love home-baked bread and would like a healthy day-to-day loaf.

Wheat & Gluten Free ✗	Lactose Free ✓	Nightshade Free ✓
Gassy Veg Free ✓	Red Meat Free ✓	

Makes 1 loaf / Ready in 3 hours or less

1 tsp yeast
500g (1lb 2oz) **Kamut flour**
½ tsp salt
1 tsp sugar
375ml (13fl oz) water
2 tbsp olive oil

In a bread machine:

- Place the yeast, Kamut flour, salt, sugar, water and olive oil in the pan of the bread machine.
- Bake on the Whole Wheat programme.

By hand:

- Put the yeast, flour, salt and sugar in a large bowl and mix together. Add the water and oil and mix again.
- Bring the dough together with your hands and knead until smooth. Cover with cling film and leave to rise for 1 hour (or until doubled in size).
- Knead again for about 5 minutes then press into a large loaf tin. Cover with cling film and leave to rise in a warm place for 25 minutes.
- Preheat the oven to 220°C/200°C Fan/425°F/Gas mark 7.
- Remove the cling film and bake for 40 minutes. Leave to cool on a wire rack.

KAMUT QUICK ROLLS

These rolls are really simple to make. Great for a lunchbox or picnic.

Wheat & Gluten Free ✕	Lactose Free ✓	Nightshade Free ✓
Gassy Veg Free ✓	Red Meat Free ✓	

Makes 8 rolls / Ready in 1 hour or less

1 egg, beaten
2 tbsp yeast
25g (1 tbsp) honey
280ml (9½fl oz) warm water
3 tbsp mild (light) olive oil, plus extra for oiling
1 tsp salt
400g (14oz) **Kamut flour**

- Mix together the egg, yeast, honey, warm water, olive oil and salt. Add the flour and start to bring together into a dough. Tip out onto a floured surface and knead until the dough is smooth.

- Divide into 8 equal balls and form into rolls. Place on an oiled or lined baking (cookie) sheet. Cover with cling film and leave to rise in a warm place for 25 minutes.
- Meanwhile, preheat the oven to 190°C/Fan 170°C/375°F/Gas mark 5.
- Bake for 15–20 minutes.

KAMUT FLATBREADS

This amazing flatbread makes an ideal lunchtime bread. It's a great way to bring bread and wheat back into your diet. For a rich, authentic flavour, leaving this bread to rise for an hour or more really adds to the depth of taste.

Wheat & Gluten Free ✗	Lactose Free ✗	Nightshade Free ✓
Gassy Veg Free ✓	Red Meat Free ✓	

Makes 6 flatbreads / Ready in 2½ hours

½ tsp yeast
200g (7oz) **Kamut flour**
50g (2oz) buckwheat flour
1 tsp sugar
½ tsp salt
½ tsp baking powder
2 tbsp (50g) **natural yogurt**
100ml (3½ fl oz) warm water
1 tbsp olive oil, plus extra for oiling

By hand:

- In a large bowl, mix together the yeast, both flours, sugar, salt and baking powder.
- Add the yogurt and warm water. Mix roughly then bring the dough together with floured hands.
- Knead vigorously, then cover the bowl with cling film and leave in a warm place for 1–2 hours.

- Knock the air out of the dough, then add the oil. Knead until the oil has been incorporated.
- Divide into 6 equal balls. Lightly grease 2 baking (cookie) sheets.
- On a floured surface, roll out each ball with a rolling pin into rough oval shapes. Transfer to the baking sheets, cover with cling film and leave to rise for about 25 minutes in a warm place.
- Preheat the grill (broiler) to the highest setting.
- Sprinkle the breads with a little water and grill for 2–3 minutes each side until brown and puffed. Wrap in a tea towel to keep warm.
- When cold these breads can be frozen and toasted directly from the freezer.

In a bread machine:

- Place the yeast, both flours, sugar, salt, baking powder, yogurt, water (cold, not warm) and olive oil in your bread machine pan.
- Use the Fast or Pizza Dough programme to make the dough. Leave in the bread machine for 1 hour after the programme has finished to allow the bread to rise.
- Remove from the bread machine and knock the air out of the dough before dividing into 6 equal balls. Lightly grease 2 baking (cookie) sheets.
- On a floured surface, roll out each ball with a rolling pin into rough oval shapes. Transfer to the baking sheets, cover with cling film and leave to rise for about 25 minutes in a warm place.
- Preheat the grill (broiler) to the highest setting.
- Sprinkle the breads with a little water and grill for 2–3 minutes each side until brown and puffed.
- Wrap in a tea towel to keep warm.
- When cold these breads can be frozen and toasted directly from the freezer.

KAMUT PIZZA DOUGH

This is a delicious and easy pizza dough that can be stretched out thin or kept fat and puffy. Also great as a garlic bread – spread with garlic, butter and Italian herbs before baking.

Wheat & Gluten Free ✕	Lactose Free ✓	Nightshade Free ✓
Gassy Veg Free ✓	Red Meat Free ✓	

Makes 1 large pizza base / Ready in 1½ hours

½ tsp yeast

300g (11oz) **Kamut flour**

1 tsp salt

200ml (7fl oz) water

1 tbsp olive oil, plus extra for oiling

By hand:

- In a large bowl, mix together the yeast, flour and salt. Add the water and oil. Knead vigorously until smooth. On a floured surface, roll out the dough to the correct size. Then transfer to an oiled baking (cookie) sheet, cover with cling film and leave to rest for 25 minutes.

In a bread machine:

- Put the yeast, flour, salt, water and oil in the bread machine pan. Use the pizza or quick dough setting.

- On a floured surface, roll out the dough to the correct size. Then transfer to an oiled baking (cookie) sheet, cover with cling film and leave to rest for 25 minutes.

- When you are ready to cook the pizza, preheat the oven to 220°C/Fan 200°C/425°F/Gas mark 7.

- Add any toppings to the pizza and bake for 10–12 minutes.

ADVENTURE RECIPES: FOOD COMBINING

EASY HOME-MADE BAKED BEANS

Wheat & Gluten Free ✓	Lactose Free ✓	Nightshade Free ✗
Gassy Veg Free ✗	Red Meat Free ✓	

Serves 2 / Ready in 15 minutes

1 × 400g (14oz) tin **haricot (navy) beans**, rinsed and drained

250ml (9fl oz) water

1 tbsp **tomato purée** (paste)

1 tbsp **tomato ketchup**

½ tsp Worcestershire sauce

½ tsp asafoetida

½ tsp **paprika**

½ tsp sugar

1 tbsp red wine vinegar

1 tsp cornflour (cornstarch), combined with a little water to make a paste

- Put the haricot (navy) beans, water, tomato purée, ketchup, Worcester-shire sauce, asafoetida, paprika, sugar and red wine vinegar in a small saucepan and bring to the boil. Reduce the heat to low and cook gently for 10 minutes.

- Stir in the cornflour (cornstarch) paste and stir well. Simmer for a further 5 minutes.

- The beans can be served immediately, but keep well in the fridge for up to 2 days.

PRAWN BIRYANI

Wheat & Gluten Free ✓	Lactose Free ✓	Nightshade Free ✗
Gassy Veg Free ✗	Red Meat Free ✓	

Serves 2 / Ready in 20 minutes

1 tsp olive oil

1 clove

1 bay leaf

1 **onion**, peeled and chopped

1 **red (bell) pepper**, deseeded and chopped

1 **garlic clove**, peeled and thinly sliced

1 red or green **chilli**, deseeded and sliced (optional)

1 tsp mild **chilli powder**

1 tsp **paprika**

¼ tsp turmeric

¼ tsp ground cumin

¼ tsp cinnamon

1 tsp salt

2 fresh **tomatoes**, roughly chopped

2 tbsp water

250g (8oz) raw king prawns (king or jumbo shrimp) (if frozen, cook for a little
    longer/defrost as per pack instructions)

250g (8oz) cooked and cooled basmati rice

1 small handful of fresh coriander (cilantro), chopped (optional)

juice of ½ lemon

lemon wedges, to serve

- In a wide, lidded frying pan (skillet), heat the oil over a medium heat. Add
  the clove and bay leaf, then the onion and red pepper. Stir, turn the heat
  to low and place the lid on the pan. Cook for 5 minutes.

- Remove the lid from the pan. Add the garlic, chilli, chilli powder, paprika,
  turmeric, ground cumin, cinnamon and salt and fry for a further minute.
  Add the chopped tomatoes and water. Replace the lid on the pan and
  cook gently for 7 minutes.

- Take the lid off and remove the clove and bay leaf. Add the prawns
  (shrimp) and cook until just pink. Add the rice, stir thoroughly and warm
  through. Finally, stir through the coriander (cilantro) and lemon juice.

- Serve with lemon wedges on the side.

BEEF BOURGUIGNON

Wheat & Gluten Free ✘	Lactose Free ✓	Nightshade Free ✓
Gassy Veg Free ✘	Red Meat Free ✘	

Serves 4 / Ready in 3–8 hours

400g (14oz) lean **casserole beef steak**, diced

100g (3½oz) **lardons** or **bacon** bits

200g (7oz) button mushrooms, washed

2 **garlic cloves**, peeled and sliced

1 medium **onion**, peeled, halved and sliced

200g (7oz) pickled **shallots**, drained

1 tsp dried thyme

2 bay leaves

2 tbsp plain (all-purpose) **flour**

400ml (14fl oz) red wine

salt and freshly ground black pepper

- Put the beef, bacon or lardons, mushrooms, garlic, onion, shallots, thyme and bay leaves into a large casserole or slow-cooker dish.

- Sprinkle on the flour and, using your hands, toss it around until everything is lightly coated.

- Next, season with salt and pepper and pour on the wine and 500ml (18fl oz) water. Give it a stir and pop on the lid.

In the oven:

- Preheat the oven to 140°C/Fan 120°C /275°F/Gas mark 1 and cook for 3 hours.

In the slow cooker:

- Cook on low for 8 hours.

SPICY BEAN BURGERS

Wheat & Gluten Free ✘	Lactose Free ✓	Nightshade Free ✘
Gassy Veg Free ✘	Red Meat Free ✓	

Serves 2 / Ready in 20 minutes, plus chilling

1 × 400g (14oz) tin **cannellini beans**, rinsed and drained

2 tbsp red pesto

75g (3oz) wholemeal (wholewheat) **breadcrumbs**

1 large egg

4 **spring onions** (scallions), trimmed and chopped

1 **garlic clove**, peeled and crushed

4 tsp olive oil (1 tsp per burger)

salt and freshly ground black pepper

- Use a potato masher to thoroughly mash the beans. Add the pesto, breadcrumbs, egg, spring onions (scallions) and crushed garlic. Add a little salt and pepper and mix well.

- Divide the mixture into 4 portions and form into balls. Place on a baking tray or plate. Squeeze the balls down with the palm of your hand to flatten and form burgers. For best results, chill at this stage for about 30 minutes (or freeze for 10 minutes) to help the burgers retain their shape.

- When you are ready to cook the burgers, heat the oil in a frying pan (skillet) over a medium heat. Add the burgers to the pan and cook for 4–5 minutes on each side until golden. Serve hot.

TRADITIONAL LAMB STEW

Wheat & Gluten Free ✓	Lactose Free ✓	Nightshade Free ✗
Gassy Veg Free ✗	Red Meat Free ✗	

Serves 6 / Ready in 4–8 hours

2 tbsp olive oil

600g (1lb 5oz) **lamb** shoulder, diced

1 **onion**, peeled and roughly chopped

3 carrots, peeled and chopped

4 celery sticks, trimmed and chopped

1 small swede, peeled and diced

2 **garlic cloves**, peeled but left whole

2 tbsp **tomato purée**

2 x 400g (14oz) tins **tomatoes**

500ml (18fl oz) **vegetable stock**

2 bay leaves

250ml (9fl oz) red wine

- Heat the oil in a large ovenproof casserole or slow-cooker dish. Add the lamb and roughly chopped onion; stir. Cook for 5 minutes until a couple of bits are burnt. Add the carrots, celery, swede and garlic. Stir and cook for another 5 minutes.

- Add the tomato purée, tinned tomatoes, stock and bay leaves. Simmer gently for 30 minutes. Add the red wine.

In the oven:

- Preheat the oven to 140°C/Fan 120°C/275°F/Gas mark 1 and cook for 4 hours.

In the slow cooker:

- Cook on low for 8 hours.

KALE SOUP WITH STILTON

Wheat & Gluten Free ✓	Lactose Free ✗	Nightshade Free ✓
Gassy Veg Free ✗	Red Meat Free ✓	

Serves 2 / Ready in 40 minutes

1 tsp olive oil

2 **leeks**, trimmed and sliced

1 potato (170g/6oz), peeled and diced

250ml (9fl oz) **vegetable stock**, fresh or made with ½ cube

150g (5oz) **kale**, shredded

30g (1oz) Stilton cheese, crumbled

1 tbsp sherry

200ml (7fl oz) skimmed (skim) **milk**

2 tbsp (30ml) double (heavy) **cream**

salt and freshly ground black pepper

- Heat the oil in a large saucepan and gently fry the leeks for 10 minutes until tender.

- Stir in the potato and add the stock. Bring to the boil, then reduce the heat and simmer gently for 15 minutes. Use a potato masher in the soup to mash the potatoes until smooth (or use a blender, if you prefer).

- Add the kale, Stilton (reserving a little for the top), sherry, milk and cream. Bring to a gentle simmer and cook for 5 minutes until the kale is tender. Season then divide between 2 bowls and top with the reserved cheese.

ONE POT MAC & CHEESE

Wheat & Gluten Free ✓	Lactose Free ✗	Nightshade Free ✓
Gassy Veg Free ✗	Red Meat Free ✓	

Serves 4 / Ready in 20 minutes

200g (7oz) buckwheat pasta

200g (7oz) butternut squash, cubed

200g (7oz) **cauliflower**, cut into small florets

2 **leeks**, trimmed and sliced

1 tsp ground nutmeg

1 tsp white pepper

1 **vegetable stock cube**, crumbled

1 bay leaf

500ml (18fl oz) **milk**

500ml (18fl oz) water

4 **garlic cloves**, crushed

150g (5oz) Cheddar cheese, grated

60g (2oz) Parmesan cheese, grated

- Take a large, shallow, lidded saucepan. Place the pasta, butternut squash, cauliflower and leeks in the pan. Add the nutmeg, pepper, stock cube and bay leaf. Pour in the milk and water and bring to the boil. Simmer for 10–12 minutes until the pasta is tender. Stir thoroughly.

- Stir in the garlic, Cheddar and Parmesan. Heat for 2 minutes, before placing the lid on the pan and leaving to rest and thicken for a further 5 minutes.

CHICKEN TAGINE

Wheat & Gluten Free ✓	Lactose Free ✓	Nightshade Free ✗
Gassy Veg Free ✗	Red Meat Free ✓	

Serves 4 / Ready in 1½ hours or less

1 tbsp olive oil

1 medium **onion**, peeled and chopped

2 tsp mild **chilli powder**

1 tsp turmeric

1 tsp ground cumin

1 × 400g (14oz) tin **chopped tomatoes**

500ml (18fl oz) **chicken stock** (made with 1 cube)

400g (14oz) potatoes, peeled (if necessary) and cut into large pieces

1 x 400g (14oz) tin **chickpeas**, rinsed and drained

60g (2oz) sultanas (golden raisins)

1 tbsp **salsa** (fresh)

1 tbsp apricot jam

4 x 125g (4oz) skinless chicken breast fillets, halved

juice of 1 lime

- Heat the oil in a large, lidded casserole dish over a low heat.

- Add the onion and fry gently for 5 minutes. Stir in the spices, then add the chopped tomatoes and stock. Bring to simmering point and cook gently for 15 minutes.

- Add the potatoes, chickpeas, sultanas, salsa and apricot jam and continue to cook for half an hour.

- Add the chicken and stir through. When the tagine just starts to bubble again, cook for 10 minutes until the chicken is just cooked through, so that the juices run clear when cut. Squeeze in the lime juice before serving.

INDEX